THE BUMP PLAN

HOLLIE GRANT

Thorsons

Thorsons
An imprint of HarperCollins*Publishers*
1 London Bridge Street
London SE1 9GF

www.harpercollins.co.uk

HarperCollins*Publishers*
Macken House, 39/40 Mayor Street Upper
Dublin 1, D01 C9W8, Ireland

First published by Thorsons 2023

10 9 8 7 6 5 4 3 2 1

While the author of this work have made every effort to ensure that the information contained in this book is as accurate and up-to-date as possible at the time of publication, medical and pharmaceutical knowledge is constantly changing and the application of it to particular circumstances depends on many factors. Therefore it is recommended that readers always consult a qualified medical specialist for individual advice. This book should not be used as an alternative to seeking specialist medical advice which should be sought before any action is taken. The author and publishers cannot be held responsible for any errors and omissions that may be found in the text, or any actions that may be taken by a reader as a result of any reliance on the information contained in the text which is taken entirely at the reader's own risk. Anywhere 'women' and 'mothers' are referred to in this book, this should be taken to include pregnant people who do not identify as women.

A catalogue record of this book is available from the British Library

ISBN 978-0-00-858919-6

Printed and bound in the UK using 100% renewable electricity at CPI Group (UK) Ltd

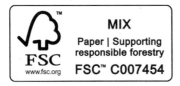

This book is produced from independently certified FSC™ paper to ensure responsible forest management.

For more information visit: www.harpercollins.co.uk/green

To Freya and Kit – may I always make you as proud as you both make me

Contents

~~~~~~

Introduction   1

Part 1: What You Need to Know   **9**
Physical activity – where do we begin?   11
Staying active during your conception,
pregnancy and postnatal journey   19
Understanding your anatomy   37

Part 2: Your Conception and Pregnancy Workouts   **59**
Let's get started   61
TTC – trying to conceive   69
Pregnancy weeks 0–6   96
Pregnancy weeks 7–12   121
Pregnancy weeks 13–19   145
Pregnancy weeks 20–27   171
Pregnancy weeks 28–33   194
Pregnancy weeks 34–40+   216

Part 3: Your Postnatal Workouts   **243**

   Birth and your body   245
   Recovery phase   261
   Postnatal phase 1   271
   Postnatal phase 2   292

Conclusion   309
Acknowledgements   311
Sources   314
Resources   323

Introduction

Welcome to *The Bump Plan* – your best friend, hype woman and survival guide to staying active during conception, pregnancy and beyond. It's the book I wish I'd read when I was pregnant with my daughter, Freya, now 4 years old, and the book I want Freya to read if she is ever pregnant. I hope it helps every person on this journey to see that staying active needn't feel like rocket science, to understand why being active can help you feel like the absolute badass that you are and to learn how staying strong will prepare you for whatever parenting throws at you (which is a lot!).

Building a strong body ahead of conception and staying active during pregnancy have vast proven health benefits, both physically and mentally. Aside from the general health gains we all make from physical activity, it also has pregnancy-specific advantages. Not only can it make being pregnant feel more comfortable and progress more smoothly, it also lessens the risk of gestational diabetes, improves cardiovascular fitness and reduces your risk of pregnancy-related blood pressure issues.[1] It can reduce labour times, improve postnatal recovery times and boost postpartum mental health.[2] There is also research to suggest that our babies themselves could benefit from having an active mother, too (how cool is that!).[3,4]

However, while pregnant with Freya I realised that exercise is a huge no man's land for pregnant women. We have a generation of women who are keen exercisers, who suddenly feel lost when they become pregnant. Around 75 per cent of pregnant women do not meet the current guidelines for activity.[5] That's a lot! Information online is often outdated and inconsistent, and many women feel scared that they might harm themselves or their babies. They are told by medical professionals that they need to stay active, yet they're not given the tools or advice as to how best to do so. So often, they do nothing, and then feel guilty about the fact they are doing nothing. It's an awful position to be in. But it is avoidable.

Postnatally, the information around physical activity isn't much better. Many women are told to wait to start exercising again until after their 6-week appointment with their doctor. Now anyone who has attended one of these appointments knows there is a lot to cover, and not a lot of time. The appointment is also, understandably, heavily focused on checking your baby is healthy, so Mum doesn't always get a look in. At my appointment, I didn't get my scar checked, despite having had an emergency Caesarean followed by sepsis. Therefore, this 6-week marker is pretty arbitrary. There is a lot you can – and should – be doing from Day 1 after giving birth that will help to improve and speed up your postnatal recovery. Therefore, more evidence-led advice needs to be shared (and don't worry – I've got you covered in Part 3).

About me

Before I go on, let me tell you a little bit about myself. Eleven years ago, I left my (short) career as an apprentice pastry chef with a celebrated chocolatier, having realised it wasn't the dream I hoped it would be. Suffering from depression, I handed in my notice and never looked back. While putting myself back together again, I took on a role as a receptionist at a Pilates studio in London. I instantly fell in love with Pilates (it really was love at first try!). I was fascinated by the focus on technique and anatomy. I loved that it was about increasing performance, rather than reducing dress size. And I was obsessed with how strong and resilient it made me feel, having spent so long feeling physically and mentally weak.

After a year of daily Pilates, the instructors at the studio gave me the push I needed to train as an instructor myself with world-renowned STOTT Pilates. I went on to become an advanced reformer and mat Pilates instructor and taught across London in studios and private residences for many years. I was promoted to head trainer at two busy Pilates studios and added a personal-training qualification to my name. Eight years ago, the opportunity arose for me to open my own studio in beautiful Parsons Green. I still consider this studio to be my first baby, and it has given me years of joy and fantastic memories and friends.

Since then, I have had a 2-year residency at the Mandarin Oriental Hotel in London, trained extensively as a pre- and post-natal fitness expert and travelled the world to teach at some of the world's most incredible hotels.

With an awareness that women needed more support to stay active on their pregnancy journey, I launched The Bump Plan Pregnancy in December 2020 – a holistic prenatal fitness plan that I filmed throughout my own pregnancy with Freya. It was created to fill a massive void, at a time when pregnant women were at home more than ever, experiencing restricted maternal care and feeling increasingly alone amid the COVID pandemic.

The Bump Plan online has now helped over 30,000 women stay active during their pregnancies. In January 2022, we launched The Bump Plan Postnatal to help women continue this journey once their babies arrive, followed by a first-of-its-kind plan for those trying to conceive (The Bump Plan TTC) in November 2022.

Over the past 11 years, I have been lucky enough to have worked with women of all ages, abilities, sizes and stages of their lives. It has been an absolute joy, and I genuinely consider myself as having one of the best jobs in the world.

Exercise and body image

Staying active during pregnancy is great for both you and your baby, but through my work I've found that exercising at this time can help to undo some of the body-image issues that plague women, too. Although I love the fitness industry, it has a dark side – one that wants women to feel inadequate, weak or out of shape. This is a side that I feel passionately needs to change. I don't want my daughter growing up in a world that tells people they must burn calories to earn food, that thinness equals success and that exercise is purely there to change the way their bodies look. And I don't want this for you, either. That said, anecdotally, with many of my clients, I have found that pregnancy is the ideal time to change any negative relationship we may have with exercise, or our bodies. It's a time when growing is seen as a positive thing; when our thoughts are about someone else's development (our babies'), rather than our own aesthetic journeys. Feeling supported at this time in your life and having the information you need to stay – or become – active is vital, and I firmly believe it can help change your relationship with your body for ever.

My aim is that this book helps you to understand why an active pregnancy is so important, showcases that it is achievable and safe, gives you the tools to exercise safely at home and helps you learn to respect your body for the rest of your life – no matter what life throws at it!

It may help to know that I've been writing this book throughout my own second pregnancy and postnatal period (I gave birth via elective Caesarean to my son Kit while finishing this book). This has given me the perfect insight into this stage of life, and a reminder of just how much exercise can improve a pregnancy experience. I'm on this journey with you, and while all our experiences will differ, I hope this shared journey is supportive for you.

How to use this book

This book is designed to support you, no matter what stage of parenting you're at – whether you're thinking about starting a family, actively trying to conceive, currently pregnant or you've joined the postpartum party (albeit less party and more constant hangover). It's never too early to start thinking about how you'll stay active during pregnancy, and it's never too late to start getting your body moving post baby.

The book is therefore split into three parts. Part 1 is the main 'information' section that'll help you understand everything you need to know about why and how you should stay active. You'll learn about the evidence supporting active pregnancies and the benefits, what the guidelines mean (and how to understand them), when you can get back to physical activity post-labour and much more. There's some anatomy, too, so you can understand what is happening to your body. And don't worry, there are some laughs thrown in there along the way. Knowledge is power, and I honestly believe that the more women understand their bodies, and what is happening to them, the less they will care about aesthetics and weight, and the more they will care about function.

Part 2 is all about the pregnancy phase of life (I also talk about trying to conceive here – or TTC). I have found that once women start trying to get pregnant, they get a little nervous about exercise and start altering how they move their bodies, or stop moving altogether. This is a totally understandable fear and, having been pregnant twice, I can completely empathise. Growing another human is one of the most incredible but daunting experiences ever, but when we are so nervous about doing anything wrong, we can sometimes fall into the trap of not doing anything at all. Staying active during pregnancy *is* safe for most women and is *so* important. The NHS defines the three main stages of pregnancy as:

- First trimester: 1–12 weeks pregnant
- Second trimester: 13–27 weeks pregnant
- Third trimester: 28–40+ weeks pregnant

In Part 2, there are eight chapters: an introduction, a chapter on trying to conceive, and six pregnancy chapters each covering half a trimester. I'll explain what's happening to your body at each step along your pregnancy journey and give you exercises tailored specifically to that stage. These exercises have been tested, and used, by thousands of women, and will help you to build a strong, resilient body to better cope with the demands of pregnancy and beyond.

In Part 3, I'll be showing you how to get back to the movement you love post-birth, safely and with respect and consideration for what your body has been through. Don't worry – there will be no 'snap-back' or 'get-your-body-back' messaging here. It is all about performance and function, not aesthetics. Part 3 will be split into three phases: Recovery, Phase 1 and Phase 2. These phases are not time-specific like the ones in Part 2. This is because we all have different pregnancies, labours and recoveries and should therefore all move through the phases at a pace that works for us. You'll learn what the guidelines are for postnatal movement, the differences between each type of birth and how they may affect you, how to support your postpartum recovery and how to gradually increase your activity until you are back to your pre-pregnancy levels (or more, should you wish).

In both Parts 2 and 3, I'll be giving you exercises that combine cardiovascular and musculoskeletal training. Throughout, I call the cardiovascular exercises 'Sweat' exercises and the musculo-skeletal exercises 'Strength' exercises. I'll be discussing what all this means and why I use this method in Part 1, but this blend of exercises and the format I'll be explaining have been tested on thousands of my own clients and are – in my opinion – the ideal combination of training for lifelong wellbeing, as well as being in line with the current guidelines from the UK Chief Medical Officers (CMOs). In each chapter, you'll also find example routines to show you how to slot the exercises into your life, a pelvic floor workout, and a supplementary section from an expert I admire on topics from nutrition to diastasis.

You'll also find pre-screening forms in the Resources section of this book (p. 323), which will help you understand if there are any health reasons that may mean you need to speak with your GP before starting your Bump Plan workouts.

I know you're going to love how this plan makes you feel. So without further chit-chat, I'll let you get stuck in. Pregnancy and parenting can be tough . . . but so are you! I hope you enjoy the book.

Part 1: What You Need to Know

Physical activity – where do we begin?

This book is designed to support you during pregnancy and post-partum, but it's important to understand what physical activity is recommended through *all* stages of life so you can understand how the advice changes when you start your parenting journey. So let's dive in …

The importance of physical activity for life

Over the last few years, there has been a huge rise in awareness around the importance of staying active, partly triggered by new guidelines and insights from the UK Chief Medical Officers (CMOs) in 2019.[1] These guidelines were incredibly important in highlighting the hugely positive effect of an active lifestyle in reducing the risk of long-term conditions *and* managing existing ones and is perfectly summed up in the words of the CMOs:

> *If physical activity were a drug, we would refer to it as a miracle cure, due to the great many illnesses it can prevent and help treat.*[2]

The data makes for stark reading: physically active people are 48 per cent less likely to suffer with depression, 25 per cent less likely to have coronary heart disease or stroke, 20 per cent less likely to develop breast cancer and 35 per cent less likely to develop type-2 diabetes. It's also thought that one in six deaths in the UK and up to 40 per cent of many long-term conditions, such as type-2 diabetes, cardiovascular diseases and some cancers, are linked to insufficient physical activity.[3] If there was a vitamin or supplement that could replicate the positive effects of physical activity, I'm sure we'd all be taking it, right?

Now the benefits of staying physically active aren't new news, but the evidence shows (time and time again) that it is vital for our long-term health. Yet for various reasons, 42 per cent of British women are not meeting the current CMO guidelines, whilst 25 per cent are considered physically inactive, and therefore not benefitting from the associated health protection.[4] And that's before we even throw the whole TTC/pregnant/postnatal journey into play.

It's therefore important that we start by looking at the guidelines for the *general adult population* – and they aren't hugely dissimilar from those we'll come on to during pregnancy and beyond. If we can enter our parenting journey already active, it can make what is to come so much easier.

According to the 2019 CMOs' physical activity guidelines, all adults should attempt to be physically active *every* day. Any activity is better than none, and more is better still. When considering our levels of physical activity, the guidelines cover three key aspects:

- **Strengthening activity.** Adults need to include activity that strengthens their musculoskeletal system at least twice per week. This should involve the major muscle groups of the upper and lower body and could take the form of weightlifting at the gym, carrying heavy shopping or activities such as racquet sports or Pilates. The aim here is to improve muscle function, bone health and balance.

- **Cardiovascular activity.** Each week, adults should aim to accumulate at least either 150 minutes of moderate intensity or 75 minutes of vigorous intensity activity, or even shorter durations of very vigorous activity or a mixture of all the above (don't worry – I'll explain intensity levels in more depth in a moment).
- **Reducing sedentary time.** Adults should aim to minimise the amount of time they spend being sedentary and, where possible, break up long periods of inactivity with at least some light physical activity.

Ok – so for some of us that might sound really convoluted or seem like a lot of activity to squeeze into a week. For others, it might seem both a reasonable and achievable commitment. And some of us might be thinking, what on earth did I just read?

Before we go any further, I think it's important that we discuss the language used when it comes to moving your body. The guidelines are for physical activity, and as I have learnt from the CEO of the Active Pregnancy Foundation Dr Marlize De Vivo, distinguishing that from terms like 'exercise' and 'sport' can make all the difference to the way we view movement. Let me explain . . .

The word 'exercise' tends to describe an activity that is planned, structured and has the intention to build strength or boost fitness – such as a group fitness class or a pre-prescribed gym routine. If we think that *only* this type of movement counts, it can feel quite restrictive – what if you can't afford these classes? Or you don't have the childcare options to go to the gym to train?

'Sport', on the other hand, is an organised form of physical activity, usually of a competitive nature and defined as a skill that is bound by rules. Sport is a fantastic way of making new friends and enjoying the associated camaraderie and collaboration. Again, however, it usually requires a specified time commitment, potentially some travel and also childcare, so it might not be accessible to all.

When we use the term 'physical activity', we are describing *any* form of bodily movement produced by skeletal muscles (the ones that connect to your bones and allow you to perform a wide range of movements) resulting in energy expenditure. It can be thought of as a very inclusive term, as it covers activities such as walking the dog, doing housework, playing with your kids and having sex, but can also include more structured movement, such as a Pilates class, or sport, such as a game of netball. Using this type of language really helps us to realise that we can get movement in so many forms – the possibilities are endless.[5]

Now let's break down the information in those guidelines above.

Strengthening activity

For a long time, cardiovascular fitness has been in the limelight when it comes to staying active, and strengthening activities haven't been prioritised in quite the same way. I believe this is partly due to the emphasis that diet culture puts on weight loss and calorie burn, which, naturally, will be higher with most cardiovascular training than with strength training (but not always). Phrases used by the fitness industry, such as, 'Go hard or go home' or, 'Sweat like a pig to look like a fox', don't help with this bias towards cardiovascular work, but we must remember that we need to be 'functionally fit' to get through life free of injury and illness. And that means we need a strong cardiovascular system (our heart, veins, arteries, capillaries) *and* a strong musculoskeletal system (bones, muscles, cartilage, ligaments, tendons, connective tissue, joints).

Muscle strengthening activities are, as the name suggests, those that build muscle strength and will load our bones, which, in turn, can make them stronger. This helps to build a body that is less likely to become injured (and an injury will usually reduce our ability to stay active) and a body that can cope with all that life (and parenting) throws at us. Therefore, we mustn't forget to prioritise strength work.

Cardiovascular activity

If we look back at the CMOs' guidelines again, we can see that we are aiming to accumulate at least 150 minutes of moderate intensity physical activity or 75 minutes of vigorous intensity activity each week. This means that we can build those minutes out of any movement we enjoy. On any given day, we might spend 15 minutes walking the dog in the morning, then do 30 minutes of hoovering at lunchtime (I love hoovering; but don't worry – I hate washing up), then go to a dance class with a friend in the afternoon or partake in some friendly bedtime action that night. All these activities can add up to a pretty substantial chunk of time and go a long way to helping us meet those recommended minutes per week. How amazing – and manageable!

Now let's look more closely at the idea of 'intensity' in its various forms.

When you move your body, it responds by increasing your heart rate, taking in more oxygen (breathing faster or harder) and potentially sweating to manage heat distribution. You can think of these effects, and your effort, as being on a sliding scale of intensity levels from 0 to 10. Let's say that 0 is when you are essentially doing nothing – no activity whatsoever. Maybe that's sleeping or sitting on the sofa watching *Bake Off* (although I get pretty animated when watching that, so I'd be at a 5).

At the other end of that scale is 10 and it's when you are working at your maximum effort. This could be near the end of a marathon, or maybe at the peak of a spin class. It's you exercising at your very hardest.

Now moderate intensity would sit at around the 6–7 mark on that scale, and you would describe it as being a bit hard, but not *very* hard. It would definitely get your heart beating faster, and your breathing rate would increase and you may well sweat, but you're not working at your very hardest. You'd still be able to talk – and that's a great way to test the intensity (we call it the 'talk test' – if you can still talk, but not quite sing, it's more than likely moderate intensity). It might involve activities such as brisk walking, riding a bike or gardening.

Vigorous intensity would sit nearer the 9 mark, and you would struggle to say more than a few words without needing to pause. It might involve activities such as running, swimming and skipping, and you'd say you were working hard.

Very vigorous intensity would describe an activity that could only be performed in short bursts and would require rest periods in between. An example would be high intensity interval training (HIIT) and it would be a 10 on your scale. You would not want to (or be able to) talk to someone.

So essentially, the terms moderate, vigorous and very vigorous simply define how hard *you* are working. And the harder you work, the fewer minutes you need to rack up.

One thing to remember is that this scale is not based on specific volumes or reps of exercise. We're not saying that maximum intensity (10 on the scale) is you at the end of doing ten burpees, and moderate intensity (6 on the scale) is you at the end of doing six burpees. This scale is based on how it feels for you alone. So moderate intensity is naturally going to look different for everyone. Someone like Serena Williams, who has a very high base-fitness level, will be able to do far more at a moderate intensity than me, for example.

Reducing sedentary time

Finally, the guidelines mention the need to reduce sedentary time. Spending long periods sitting, even if you're managing to meet the guidelines for cardiovascular activity, has been shown to be harmful to health, so an attempt at reducing this is of great importance. If time spent sitting is unavoidable because of work, social or mobility reasons, break these periods up with light activity.

So if we revisit the guidelines for the general adult population one last time, we can see that:

- all activity counts – so you may as well do what you enjoy
- you must include both cardiovascular *and* muscle strengthening activities
- you should try to be active every day, if possible, and avoid long periods of sitting.

We can also see that none of this has to cost any money, it won't necessarily require childcare and no special equipment is needed. Be creative with how you move, and you'll find that getting in the recommended amounts of physical activity is far more manageable than you might have thought.

Staying active during your conception, pregnancy and postnatal journey

So you're thinking of trying to conceive (often referred to as 'TTC')...

Well firstly, I'm sending you lots of strength and hope. For some of you, this may be your first attempt, for others, maybe you already have children, and I know there will be some of you who have been here before but have yet to bring home a little one. Whatever stage you are at, I'm thinking of you, as it isn't always straightforward, but it's definitely one hell of a journey. To those of you who are trying to concieve after a previous loss, I know it can be a really difficult experience and I hold you all in my thoughts. It may be helpful to know that there is a whole TTC community out there, so for those of you who find strength in numbers, and feel you need a support network, searching for TTC online could give you just that.

Now if you haven't yet actually started trying, and are just flirting with the idea, can I kindly but strongly suggest you start getting your physical activity levels up to the current guidelines (unless of course there is a medical reason why you can't). For most people, it is so much easier to do this pre-TTC and pre-pregnancy than when they are in the thick of it. It's also a great time to get active, as there are no pregnancy-specific limitations on you yet (which there can be at certain stages of the journey to come), so you can run, jump, skip, crunch and dive as much as you wish at this point, unless you have been told otherwise by your GP.

Once you are formally TTC, you enter somewhat of a grey area. There are currently, in the UK, no official physical activity guidelines for pre-conception. This is partly due to a lack of large-scale, quality research in this area, but this will hopefully change with time. The lack of evidence means it's an area that's rife with conflicting and confusing advice from unofficial sources, and is one of the reasons why women start questioning their levels of physical activity when TTC, particularly if they aren't successful straight away. They will often cut things like exercise out, in the hope that this may speed up conception, even though there's no real evidence to suggest that this would be helpful.

The lack of official physical activity guidelines therefore leaves you with two options: you can continue to follow the CMOs' adult guidelines for physical activity, or you can follow the CMOs' guidelines for pregnant women.

Now I know this may not sound particularly helpful, but it allows you to make the decision you feel most comfortable with, using the evidence you have in front of you. As I have mentioned, so many women cease physical activity when they start trying to conceive, often because they've heard someone's uneducated advice or a rumour, and that is such a shame. But the health benefits of staying active apply to you even when you are trying to conceive.

Research to date

We've established that research into staying active when TTC is scant, but what do the studies that *are* out there suggest? Well, it really is a conflicting space at present. Unexplained infertility remains of widespread concern globally and getting to the root of it may take some time. There are so many factors at play when it comes to fertility/infertility, such as BMI, stress levels, physical activity levels, diet and age, and isolating them in order to run studies that will produce accurate research can be tricky.

There is some evidence to support the theory that 'moderate exercise benefits fertility, and that high intensity and high frequency exercise may adversely affect fertility'.[6] What research there is has shown that those who take part in regular moderate intensity physical activity have higher rates of pregnancy and healthier ones.[7] Other research points towards the benefit of physical activity alongside weight loss in those with higher BMIs, and suggests that conception can take longer for those on either end of the BMI spectrum.[8]

I personally used the CMOs' guidelines for pregnancy when I was trying to conceive (I'll be taking you through these shortly), which meant that I was getting into the habit of moving my body in the way I would need to if I were to get pregnant. It also meant that I was working at moderate rather than high intensity. I must stress, though, that this was my personal choice, based on the limited research out there at the time. It was also in the context of a simple conception journey; I haven't struggled with any fertility issues in the past, and have no health concerns, so I had no constraints with my decisions. You may choose to follow a different path, and that is totally acceptable, particularly if you have any fertility concerns or have suffered a loss. We all make decisions based on what feels right for us, and that is so important.

You will notice that in the TTC workout section of the book (in Part 2) there is a heavy focus on musculoskeletal strength-based exercises (termed 'Strength' exercises) that will help to ensure that your body is strong and resilient ahead of pregnancy. With the cardiovascular-based exercises (termed 'Sweat' exercises), you can choose to train at either moderate or high intensity. (Should you need a reminder, do pop back to pp. 14–17 for the lowdown on intensity levels and the difference between cardiovascular training and musculoskeletal strength training.)

The NHS state that 'most couples (about 84 out of every 100) will get pregnant within a year if they have regular sex and don't use contraception'.[9] If you are concerned that it is taking you longer to conceive than you feel it should, please do speak to your doctor. If you are taking part in fertility treatment or assisted conception, please do head to p. 92 to learn more about the guidance for physical activity as you go through this process.

I am aware that this is not a clear-cut do-this-don't-do-that explanation for staying active while TTC, but, hopefully, it gives you an insight based on the official information that is out there. I would say that unless you have previously struggled to conceive or are worried about your fertility, there is no reason to cease exercising completely. And if you are worried that your physical activity levels are negatively affecting your fertility, please speak to your doctor.

I'm pregnant – now what?

Over the past 11 years, I have seen a huge shift in the way women view physical activity, how they train their bodies and their reasons for wanting to take part in sport. For the most part, this has been a positive step, and it is so inspiring to see women's fitness taking centre stage.

For many women, being active is a huge part of their identity and, often, their mental health support plan, yet I see a lot of them stop when they see those two blue lines. Many are nervous to train too hard, or worried that they may harm their babies, so they completely stop the activities they used to enjoy. I can understand why you might think that exercising could be harmful to your growing baby – after all, it can be strange to think of a foetus the size of a blueberry bouncing around while you jog – but let me be clear: the official advice is *not* to stop moving.

Unlike with TTC, there is a vast body of evidence out there to show that staying active during pregnancy is one of the most important things you can do to support your physical and mental health. If you are a healthy woman, experiencing an uncomplicated pregnancy, there is no reason not to continue with the movement you did pre-pregnancy – just with a few tweaks to your training (which I will come to in a moment).

Staying active during pregnancy has been shown to reduce your risk of gestational diabetes (diabetes that develops in pregnancy) and high blood pressure problems, improve cardiovascular fitness, help manage pregnancy weight gain, improve sleep and boost your mental health.[10] And all physical activity counts towards these incredible health benefits, too, so literally every minute you move your body contributes.

It's also important to note that there is no evidence of any relationship between being physically active and preterm birth, babies who are either small or large for gestational age or other complications for a newborn baby when healthy women engage in low–moderate activities. I mention this because I hear it as a common concern from women, and one of the main reasons they stop exercising, but I'll say it again for those at the back: there is no evidence of any harm to your baby.

The current guidelines for physical activity in pregnancy

At the time of writing, the current physical activity guidelines during pregnancy from the UK Chief Medical Officers are as follows:

> *Healthy pregnant women, experiencing an uncomplicated pregnancy, should aim to accumulate at least 150 minutes of moderate intensity physical activity per week, and include muscle strengthening activities twice a week.*[11]

These guidelines are really similar to the ones we read about for the general adult population (see p. 13). This is because we essentially want women to continue to move their bodies throughout pregnancy, as they did beforehand.

So we are still aiming for 150 minutes of physical activity with muscle strengthening activities included. The only real difference between the general adult guidelines and the pregnancy ones, is the *intensity* – because during pregnancy, most of us will be keeping our intensity level at 'moderate'. However, guidance produced by the WHO (World Health Organization) in 2020 says:

'Women who, before pregnancy, habitually engaged in vigorous intensity aerobic activity, or who were physically active, can continue these activities during pregnancy and the postpartum period.'

Let's just have a quick recap of some of the key language and terminology (see pp. 12–17 for more detail):

- **Physical activity.** Any form of bodily movement produced by skeletal muscles that results in energy expenditure.
- **Moderate intensity.** An activity that increases the heart and breathing rate, but still allows you to talk.
- **Muscle strengthening activities.** These strengthen the musculoskeletal system, involving major muscle groups of the upper and lower body. The aim here is to improve muscle function, bone health and balance.

So now you know what the guidelines mean for you and, hopefully, you're starting to form a picture of how you can achieve or at least build up to them. Now what else do you need to know?

Functionally fit

The guidelines specifically mention muscle strengthening exercises. This is because we want mothers to be 'functionally fit'.

Being a parent is one of the most physically demanding things I've ever done (and that's coming from someone who once ran/walked/cried my way through seven marathons in seven consecutive days). It requires constant lifting (your baby out of their cot), squatting (during labour or later, to get down to their level), hip hinging (you'll be wiping a lot of puréed peas off the floor) and endurance (for all that rocking to sleep). It will challenge your body to withstand stress positions, with limited sleep and rest, at all hours of the day and night. And babies only get heavier. So what we want are mothers that are not only cardiovascular fit, but who also have the muscle strength and endurance to effectively perform the activities they need to – and that's what we mean by functionally fit.

Ever heard the phrase 'Use it or lose it'? Well, there is some truth to this. So to get strong from a musculoskeletal point of view, some of the activity you do each week needs to challenge your muscles, all across the body. To put it simply, you don't want to be spending all 150 minutes of the activity guidelines doing one specific form of cardiovascular fitness (jogging, for example) and nothing else. Yes, you would get better at jogging, but that's not going to help you when you're holding a sleeping baby and your arms feel like they might drop off.

That's why you'll notice that Part 2 includes both Sweat and Strength exercises. The Sweat exercises will target your cardio-vascular fitness, while the Strength ones will target your musculoskeletal strength. Simple, really.

For those of you who were already active before pregnancy, your goal is to continue with the type of activity you did previously (with a few tweaks, which we'll come to soon). If, however, you were inactive, it's time to start moving. Start gradually (with, say, 20-minute workouts max) and build up as you feel ready. And it is never too late in your pregnancy to start.

So is there anything I *can't* do?

This is one of the questions I am asked most when it comes to prenatal fitness. Personally, I prefer to discuss what pregnant women *can* do, as it can feel like there are a lot of can'ts when we're pregnant. However, there are a few activities that aren't advised. Some may seem like common sense, but let's discuss them anyway:

Don't bump the bump

Essentially, you want to avoid impact to your bump as much as possible, so this would rule out contact sports such as rugby or judo, and activities that may involve an increased risk of falling, such as horse riding or skiing.

Don't scuba dive

The baby hasn't the necessary protection against decompression sickness and gas embolism.

Don't exercise at heights over 2500m above sea level

This would put you and your baby at risk of altitude sickness, and risk lowering uterine blood flow.

Don't lie flat on your back

Lying flat on your back for too long is not advised, particularly after the first trimester, due to the increased risk of reduced cardiac output and the potential for orthostatic hypotensive disorder or supine hypotensive disorder (see pp. 151–152). This is where the weight of your uterus presses on major blood vessels and can affect your blood pressure. Try to find alternative positions where possible or use a wedge or pillows to bring yourself into an incline position instead.

While it may sound obvious, if you feel unwell or are in pain during an activity, stop immediately and speak to your midwife or doctor if you are concerned. You must also stop exercising and contact your doctor if you notice any of the following[12]:

> - Vaginal bleeding
> - Abdominal pain
> - Regular painful contractions
> - Amniotic fluid leakage
> - Dyspnea (shortness of breath) before exertion
> - Dizziness
> - Headache
> - Chest pain
> - Muscle weakness affecting balance
> - Calf pain or swelling

It's important that you stay hydrated when exercising, don't allow yourself to get too hot and stop at any point if something doesn't feel right. But otherwise, you can jiggle, wriggle, dance and move to your heart's content.

Is there anyone who *shouldn't* be physically active in pregnancy?

You may have noticed that the CMOs' guidelines are for healthy pregnant women with uncomplicated pregnancies. But what does that mean, and how can you tell if you fit into that category? Well, this is where 'contraindications' come in.

There is a subset of women for whom being physically active (or altering their physical activity levels) is contraindicated, due to either pre-existing or pregnancy-specific health conditions. Contraindications themselves fall into two categories: absolute contraindications and relative contraindications:

- **Absolute contraindications** are conditions where MVPA (moderate to vigorous intensity physical activity) would not be recommended. This is because the risks outweigh the possible benefits and could cause adverse effects for mother and/or foetus. Usual activities of daily living may continue.

- **Relative contraindications** are conditions where the current guidelines for activity may not be suitable for the individual, and a discussion with their healthcare provider is advised before participation. The benefits, and risks, of physical activity should be evaluated with a professional, and modifications may need to be made (rather than a complete avoidance of physical activity).

So essentially, if you are aware or suspect that exercise might be contraindicated for you, it is imperative that you speak to your healthcare provider about your physical activity levels. They will explain the risks and benefits, and help you to formulate a plan moving forwards.

As the evidence base grows, there are changes in the list of contraindications from time to time, so it's always worth speaking to your GP if you are unsure. It's also important to note that your health can vary during pregnancy, so while you may not start out with any contraindications, it's worth revisiting the list if your health changes at all. The list of contraindications at the time of writing can be seen below[13]:

Absolute contraindications

- Severe respiratory diseases (e.g. chronic obstructive pulmonary disease, restrictive lung disease, cystic fibrosis, asthma, shortness of breath, chronic coughing and chest tightness)
- Severe acquired or congenital heart disease with exercise intolerance
- Uncontrolled or severe arrhythmia
- Placental abruption
- Vasa previa
- Uncontrolled type-1 diabetes
- Intrauterine growth restriction (IUGR)
- Active preterm labour (i.e. regular and painful uterine contractions before 37 weeks of pregnancy)
- Severe pre-eclampsia
- Cervical insufficiency

Relative contraindications

- Mild respiratory disorders (see above)
- Mild congenital or acquired heart disease
- Well-controlled type-1 diabetes
- Mild pre-eclampsia
- Preterm premature rupture of membranes (PPROMs)
- Placenta previa after 28 weeks
- Untreated thyroid disease
- Symptomatic, severe eating disorders
- Multiple nutrient deficiencies and/or chronic undernutrition
- Moderate to heavy smoking (>20 cigarettes per day) in the presence of comorbidities

Hopefully, this has helped you to see that – for most women – staying active during pregnancy is achievable, manageable and a really positive part of their journey. While there's no question that life can throw you curveballs (pregnancy symptoms, work and life stress, childcare issues), I want you to know that any movement you can include in your week will make a huge difference to your physical and mental health, your feelings of empowerment and your experience of pregnancy and parenting. You have it within you, and I'm here to hold your hand along the way.

Getting back to movement postnatally

Once you've had your baby, everything changes. It's a life-altering, earth-shattering experience. You are now a parent (maybe not for the first time), responsible for a small helpless human. I could fill many books with stories about the ginormous effect this has on every aspect of your life, but I will stick to the physical activity part here.

I want to start by acknowledging that everyone's birth experience will be different. So I will try hard to remain impartial, and not allow my own experiences to impact my writing. I will therefore often stick to the official guidelines, rather than anecdotal advice. But I do feel it's important to acknowledge that while guidelines are built on large bodies of stats and evidence, these won't always reflect individual experience.

Essentially, what I am trying to say here (maybe not that eloquently) is that some births are amazing, and some (like mine with Freya) are hard. Some women enter parenthood full of joy and positivity, feeling totally at ease with life with a newborn. Others enter it exhausted, traumatised and with at least an undertone of anxiety. So please don't panic if you see something in these pages and think, I just don't think I could do that yet. Recovery times will vary, as will the amount of support or childcare you have and your mental health. You do what you can, when you can and if it feels right for you, and don't worry about fitting perfectly into the guidelines. They are, as the name suggests, simply for guidance.

When it comes to moving your body postnatally, compared to prenatally, the concerns are usually slightly different. Anecdotally, many of the reasons I hear from women for being nervous of physical activity during pregnancy are down to fear around their baby's health and safety. They are often worried they might harm their baby, or 'do something wrong'.

Postnatally, though, women often become concerned for themselves – worried they might hurt themselves or cause long-lasting damage. There are also some women who simply jump back into doing too much too soon, and don't fully appreciate the huge changes their bodies have been through. The snap-back culture we live in, sadly, doesn't help, but it's important to focus on you, and not compare yourself to anyone else.

I feel it's important, then, to discuss what has happened physically during birth (this comes in Part 3), what the warning signs are that you may be overdoing it and how to know when it's the right time to move on to something more challenging. If you have all the information in front of you, and you learn to listen to your body (easier said than done, I know), you will be more confident as you progress.

So let's start with what the CMOs have to say about physical activity for women after childbirth.

As well as the vast array of general health gains that physical activity affords the general adult population:

... the benefits of physical activity in the postpartum period (up to one year) were identified as a reduction in depression; improved emotional wellbeing; improved physical conditioning; and reduction in postpartum weight gain and a faster return to pre-pregnancy weight.[14]

For those who were active before labour, I also feel that getting back to movement can be a powerful personal experience. I hear from so many Bump Plan members who say they cried with happiness the first time they got back on their mat after having their babies, as it signalled moving forwards and a return to some normality. It can remind you that while your baby is undoubtedly important, so are you! So don't underestimate the mental health boost to be gained from simply carving out some time to focus on your wellbeing.

The actual guidelines for postnatal women are again to gradually build back up to accumulating 150 minutes of moderate intensity physical activity every week and build back up to muscle strengthening exercises twice per week. I talk about *building back up* because you are not expected to meet these guidelines the week after you've given birth. Depending on your delivery and how you're feeling, it's about starting gradually and increasing as you feel able to do so.

That said, the guidelines are important because, for a long time, women felt they needed to wait until their 6–8-week check-up with their doctor before doing *any* physical activity, even if they felt physically able to. Most mums will, hopefully, get the green light at this appointment, but there are things you can do even before then. The key here is to start light activity as soon as *you* feel comfortable to get moving and build up gradually.

Now what this looks like in one person's mind, might be very different in another's, and it highlights how everyone's postnatal recovery will be very different. This is why putting timelines on postnatal recovery just doesn't work. Let's take two examples of new mothers:

Mother 1 was super active during pregnancy and continued to run right up until she gave birth. She had a smooth vaginal delivery at home, and has since had a lot of support with family and friends able to step in. She felt comfortable going on long walks early on and returned to running within 4 months of having her baby.

Mother 2 struggled to stay active during pregnancy due to a relative contraindication. She then had a traumatic Caesarean birth, and has had limited support at home with no family nearby. She is anxious as to what is safe for her to do, still feels discomfort around her scar and has very little energy or time to commit to her own wellbeing.

You might identify with elements of both women's experiences. The point is, we are not all the same, and we do not need to adhere to anyone else's timeframe. It really comes down to listening to your body and only progressing at a speed that feels comfortable for you, knowing the warning signs that you are overdoing it (see p. 36) and seeking help from a specialist pelvic health physiotherapist if you feel you need additional support.

The first few weeks

I'll be going into this in a lot more depth in Part 3, but once you have had your baby, there is a lot you can do, even while sat on the sofa feeding them. This is about rehabilitating your body and giving it the tools to support itself before you start increasing your activity levels.

Pelvic floor exercises

No matter how you gave birth, these can be started as soon as it is comfortable (and as long as there is no catheter in place) and can make a huge difference to the tone and function of your pelvic floor. Remember that it went through a lot during pregnancy, so even those who had a Caesarean birth need to give their pelvic floor some love.

Gentle stretching

Cuddling, feeding, changing, carrying are all incredible jobs, but they can become pretty uncomfortable after a while and can lead to some tension areas. Gentle stretching, particularly in positions you aren't spending much time in, can really improve how your body feels from day to day.

Breathwork

Not only does breathwork help to calm down the nervous system (and Lord knows, we need this as new parents), but it also starts to stimulate the core and pelvic floor and improve breathing technique.

Deep core activation

Your abdominals have stretched during pregnancy to allow your uterus the room to grow with your baby. Introducing deep core activation early on can help bring back strength and tone to the core.

Now I'll be teaching you how to introduce these activities into your recovery in Part 3, and I'll also be discussing how the way you gave birth may dictate what feels right and at what stage.

Warnings signs that you may be overdoing it

If you experience any of the following, you may be overdoing it and need to contact your doctor immediately:

> - Very heavy bleeding, like soaking through more than one pad in an hour or noticing large blood clots; bleeding in the first 2–6 weeks postnatally is normal, but if you notice it gets heavier or changes colour after your workouts, it may mean you need to scale back the intensity
> - A red or swollen leg that feels warm or painful to touch
> - A bad headache that doesn't get better after taking medication, or one that affects your vision
> - A fever of 38°C or higher
> - An incision that isn't healing

And please call 999 (or your country's emergency number) immediately if you experience:

- chest pain
- trouble breathing or shortness of breath
- seizures.

In Part 3, we'll talk more about what the recovery journey is going to look like, and how this might differ, depending on labour. I'll give you lots of guidance on exercises, techniques and skills that will help you get back to smashing fitness goals, or simply feeling more comfortable in your body. For now, though, stay with me, as we move on to discuss anatomy and what actually happens to our bodies as they go through this experience.

Understanding your anatomy

Before we get stuck into your pregnancy and postnatal recovery exercises and advice, I think it's important to give you a summary of what's actually going on inside your body. As you know, hundreds of systems work simultaneously to ensure its smooth functioning; in fact, the human body is so complex, varied and constantly adapting that we could discuss anatomy all day, or all week, and still only scratch the surface. What I hope to achieve here, though, is to give you an understanding of the cardiovascular and musculoskeletal systems that will enable you to practise your exercises with good form, acknowledge the changes that occur during pregnancy and postpartum and really give you a feel for how your body works.

With that in mind, let's jump in and learn about the body.

The cardiovascular system

We've talked a lot so far about cardiovascular fitness, so it makes sense to start with the cardiovascular system – a vitally important part of who we are.

The cardiovascular system (sometimes called the blood circulatory system) is responsible for delivering nutrients and oxygen to all the cells in our bodies (called cellular respiration), to help them convert energy from the food we eat into a usable form. It does this by forcing the blood (which is carrying said nutrients and oxygen) around the body for use, and bringing it back to the lungs to be 'refuelled'. The cardiovascular system is made up of the heart and the blood vessels that make their way through the body.

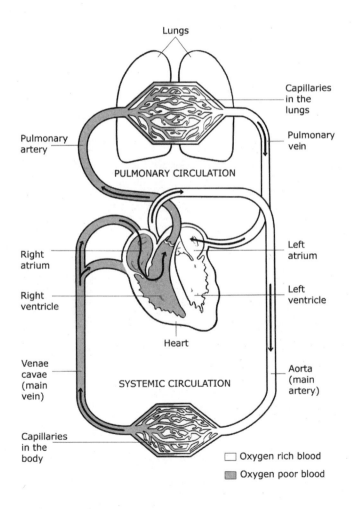

The heart is separated into two sides (left and right) by a wall of muscle and tissue called the septum and has four chambers – two atria and two ventricles. The heart is around the size of a fist, and it's responsible for pumping about 5 litres of blood around the body, all the time. It is an involuntary muscle, meaning it does its job automatically.

The flow of blood around the body can be imagined as one big chain of events, orchestrated by the heart. If you look at the diagram opposite, you can see the heart at the centre (in the body, it sits at the front of your chest, just slightly left of your breastbone) with the blood vessels extending from it to the entire body.

With each heartbeat, blood is passed from the heart, around the body and back again. Let's look at this in one cycle, starting with oxygenated blood in the left atrium:

- As the heart relaxes after a heartbeat, the blood moves from the left atrium into the left ventricle.
- With the next contraction of the heart, the blood is forced out of the ventricle into the aorta, the main artery away from the heart. The aorta splits off into smaller and smaller arteries, via which the blood heads off to deliver oxygen, nutrients and other important materials to the cells, swapping them for waste products and carbon dioxide.
- This blood is now collected up by the veins and taken back to the heart (as it is now deoxygenated and this needs to be rectified) and into the right atrium.
- Again, as the heart relaxes, the blood flows from the atrium into the right ventricle, and with the next heart contraction it is pumped away from the heart, to be taken to the lungs and into the pulmonary artery.

- The pulmonary artery branches into smaller arteries and capillaries, which, eventually, end up passing through the lungs, with the blood depositing its carbon dioxide and collecting new oxygen. This carbon dioxide is breathed out and oxygen is breathed back in, ready to be used. The freshly oxygenated blood is then carried via the pulmonary veins, back to the heart and into the left atrium, ready to perform this cycle all over again.

This beautiful, automatic process is incredibly important in keeping the cells of the body alive. A healthy, working, cardiovascular system is one of the biggest gifts there are, and we know that certain forms of activity can help to strengthen it. How incredible is that?

Now throw pregnancy into the mix and you'll have a whole new appreciation of just how amazing your cardiovascular system is, because it starts to adapt as early as 5 weeks in.

What happens to my cardiovascular system during pregnancy?

Pregnancy is associated with significant changes to the cardiovascular system, and from very early on. These changes are made to meet the new, greater demands on the mother of growing another human, and to help support the placenta as it supports the baby.

Here is a list of all these incredible adaptations – in no particular order . . . because they are all incredible (seriously, how amazing are we?).

- **Vasodilation of the systemic vasculature takes place.** This means that the blood vessels that take blood away from the heart, around the body and back to the heart, dilate (get wider) and allow more blood to flow through them. This happens as early as 5 weeks' gestation.

- **Cardiac output increases.** Cardiac output can be defined as the volume (in litres) of blood your heart can pump in 1 minute. This will increase throughout pregnancy and by week 24 it can be increased by up to 45 per cent in a singleton pregnancy.[15] It's calculated as:

Heart rate (beats per minute) × stroke volume (ml per beat)

- **Blood pressure decreases.** This happens particularly in the first and second trimesters, but it increases again to non-pregnant levels in the third trimester.[16]
- **Heart rate increases.** This can be by as much as 10–20 beats per minute (or a 20–25 per cent increase) by the third trimester.
- **Stroke volume increases.** Stroke volume is the amount of blood pumped out of the left ventricle of the heart with each beat.
- **Blood volume, plasma volume and red-blood-cell mass increase.** The blood volume can increase by around 50 per cent by the end of your third trimester. That's a lot more fluid in your body.[17]
- **Temporary remodelling of the heart's structure.** It is thought that the increased demand on the heart causes an increase in dimensions of the ventricular cavity. Your heart literally changes shape!

With all these changes going on, maintaining a functional, healthy cardiovascular system before, during and after pregnancy is therefore vital for the health of both mother and baby. Cardiovascular fitness may feel different during pregnancy (you may feel out of breath more easily, for example), but your body is adapting in ways that are beyond mind-blowing, and is doing so to give you as smooth a pregnancy as possible.

The musculoskeletal system

We have spoken already about the fact that we should all be including muscle strengthening activities into our weekly routine and how this can benefit the musculoskeletal system. But let's discuss what this system is exactly, and why it's so important.

The musculoskeletal system is made up of bones, ligaments, tendons, cartilage, joints and muscles that, together, create the framework of the body. Its main responsibilities are to support the body and allow it to move, and to protect vital organs. The skeleton itself is the main storage system for calcium and phosphorous, and plays a role in blood production and fat storage.

If we further break down the musculoskeletal system into the skeletal and muscular systems, you'll see how the two work so closely together.

The skeletal system

Imagine a skeleton, if you will. You'll hopefully be able to picture a skull, spine, ribcage, pelvis and limbs. Notice how it is all connected and everything has its own place. Viewed in this way, without skin or organs, we can see that the skeleton gives our bodies their distinctive shape and structure – it essentially gives us a home, housing our vital organs, and it's been made in a way that allows movement.

Our bones have their own role in regulating mineral balance in the bloodstream (they store minerals, so they can be released or reabsorbed, as and when needed), they store fat for desperate times of starvation and they play a role in blood-cell production. They are incredibly important in their own right, but for the purposes of this book, play a vital role in posture, movement and support.

The muscular system

Without the muscular system, we would look just like the skeleton I asked you to envisage above. It provides support to the joints, helps create movement of the body and provide stability and stillness when needed.

Our bones connect to each other at joints (otherwise, we would simply fall apart). Each joint has its own function, its own role and its own range of movement, as facilitated by the muscular system. The following helpers show up at joints:

- **Muscles.** Skeletal muscles move joints (or prevent movement). They are responsible for voluntary movement of the body such as kicking, jumping, running. Our central nervous system sends messages to the muscles to tell them to contract at a certain rate, and this allows them to have an effect (or sometimes prevent an effect) on the movement of the body. An example of this would be during a bicep curl. The bicep muscle is told to activate, it contracts and shortens and flexes the elbow.

- **Tendons.** Tendons connect muscles to bone. They are formed of a tough, flexible band of fibrous connective tissue that forms a bridge between the bone itself and the muscle. They help to manage the forces created by the bone and muscles' actions, to prevent injury to the muscle itself.
- **Ligaments.** These connect bone to bone, to form a joint. Made of strong, fibrous connective tissue, they help to protect a joint from dislocation and prevent movements that the joint shouldn't be doing.
- **Cartilage.** Cartilage is another tough, smooth type of connective tissue that covers the surface of joints and reduces friction between two bones (acting like a cushion). It can also hold bones together or create whole parts of us, such as the external part of our ears.

What happens to my musculoskeletal system during pregnancy?

During pregnancy, the most obvious change for most of us is going to be the gradual (or what for some feels like the rapid) development of a pregnancy 'bump'. Our uterus, initially nestled low down in the pelvic cavity, will increase in size and grow upwards and outwards as your baby grows to form the tell-tale sign of a bump.

As the uterus grows, various organs are moved, squashed, rotated and essentially forced to make room for it. This has several effects, such as more frequent urination (your bladder is squashed and can hold less), an increased likelihood of heartburn (your uterus presses up into your stomach), reducing how much you can eat at meals and many more.

I'll be going into more depth on these symptoms and effects in Part 2, but for the purposes of this section, I want to talk about what this growing bump does to your posture, muscles and joints, focusing on three muscle groups that come into their own in pregnancy: the abdominal wall, the pelvic floor and the glutes.

The abdominal wall

Now that we understand a little more about how the musculo-skeletal system works, we can see the huge amount of support our skeleton gets from joints and muscles. The tension we hold or create with our muscles helps to either move us or prevent movement. We also know that the area that goes through some of the biggest changes in the body is the abdominal area – where we develop our bump. It's safe to presume, therefore, that the abdominal muscles are going to be altered as your bump gets bigger because your uterus sits beneath the abdominal wall. What do you think happens to them?

Well, let's first look at what the abdominals are and what they do.

We often think of the abdominals as being just the sexy 'six-pack' muscles, but they are so much more than that. Aside from creating and/or preventing movement, the abdominals also do the following:

- They protect your internal abdominal organs (like your intestines and liver) from external trauma. Think about when someone tries to prod or punch you in the tummy, you may notice you tense your abdominal wall for protection.
- They assist in breathing. Your abdominals relax when you inhale, to manage the change in intra-abdominal pressure, but can help with a forced expiration (for example, when blowing out a candle) when they contract.
- They help with voiding activities such as coughing, vomiting, defecating, urinating, and giving birth (hooray!).

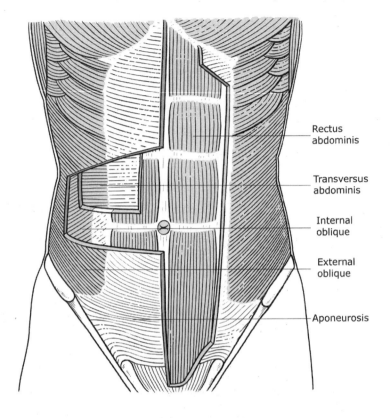

The abdominal wall consists of the rectus abdominis, external obliques, internal obliques and transversus abdominis.

Rectus abdominis

This is also known as the six-pack, but let me make it very clear: actually showcasing a six-pack requires a low level of body fat, not necessarily strength in this muscle. I have always said that aggressively aiming for a six-pack is a waste of the short time we have on this earth, and a lot comes down to genetics anyway. I'd focus on global physical strength and function, rather than homing in on this one showboater (can you tell I've never had a six-pack myself?).

Now the rectus abdominis is actually a pair of muscles that run vertically alongside each other, from the pubic bone at the front of the pelvis to the middle of the ribcage, separated by a piece of connective tissue, the linea alba, which gives us the distinctive vertical indent in a six-pack.

What is it responsible for?

- When the pelvis is fixed (i.e. stays still), these muscles create flexion of the trunk (for example, when performing a sit-up).
- When the ribcage is fixed (i.e. stays still), these muscles create a posterior tilt of the pelvis (for example, tucking your bottom under).

External obliques

The external obliques are the most superficial of our lateral abdominals (they sit closest to the skin) and can be thought of as making up the sides of the trunk. They come from the sides of ribs five to 12 and run inwards, towards the linea alba and sternum, and downwards, towards the hip bones and pubic bone. They are occasionally (and quite hilariously) called the 'penis pointers', but you can also imagine them running in a line that mimics you putting your hands into your coat pockets.

What are they responsible for?

- They can pull the chest cavity downwards – compressing the ribcage.
- If both sides of the external obliques contract, they flex the trunk (bringing the ribcage down towards the pelvis).
- If one side contracts, it can laterally flex the trunk (bending you to the side).
- They play a role in rotation of the trunk.

Internal obliques

The internal obliques also make up the sides of the trunk (think the space between the ribcage and hip bones, where you might put your hands on your hips in frustration). The fibres run in the opposite direction to the external obliques. They begin in the lower back and around the hip bone, and run up and in towards the lower ribs, and also into the linea alba and the pubic bone.

What are they responsible for?

- If both sides of the internal obliques contract, they flex the trunk (bringing the ribcage down towards the pelvis).
- If one side contracts, it can laterally flex the trunk (bending you to the side).
- They assist forced expiration by pulling down on the lower ribs, as in coughing, for example.
- They play a role in rotation of the trunk.

Transversus abdominis

In my world, this is actually the sexy muscle and I will talk about it a lot in this book. While we should never put one muscle on a pedestal, I'm going to with this one because it is your best friend during pregnancy and beyond!

This muscle extends around your lower back, hip bones and lower ribs, and comes into the linea alba and pubic bone at the front. The muscle runs transversally (hence the name) wrapping around your trunk, very much like a corset.

You'll notice that many of the Strength exercises in Part 2 focus on encouraging the transversus abdominis to stay strong, so that it can support your lower back muscles in stabilising and supporting the pelvis and lower back, while your abdominals adapt to pregnancy.

What is it responsible for?

- It increases fascial tension.
- It creates a corset effect that narrows the waist and flattens the abdomen, which has a stabilising effect on the trunk.
- It stabilises the pelvis and lower back ahead of movement.

The muscles in the abdominal wall play an incredibly important role during pregnancy. The uterus sits behind your abdominal muscles, within your abdominal cavity, and, as we've seen, it gets bigger during pregnancy, as your baby grows. Depending on where the abdominals lie (at the various stages of pregnancy) and the direction of the muscle fibres, these muscles either stretch and lengthen or they move apart to allow growth. This is an incredibly clever adaptation and allows your body to soften and adapt to your growing bump, rather than working against it.

However, there will, of course, be a change in how the body moves and functions when there is a change to the integrity and length of the muscles, and therefore some women may notice a change in their posture during pregnancy – most notably to the shape of the lower spine and an occasional increase in lower back tension or tightness. To appreciate why this can happen, we need to understand muscle imbalances.

In a very simplistic way, when we think of a joint, we can think of two bones that are next to each other being held together by ligaments and controlled by surrounding muscles. Let's imagine that only two muscles are working on the joint (usually, there are many more): one creates flexion (bending) and one creates extension (straightening back out). We need both muscles to be strong and good at their jobs for the joint to be able to both flex and extend. We also need the muscles to be equally strong at rest, so that the tug of war that occurs (one muscle trying to flex the joint and one trying to extend it) balances out and we get stillness (or neutral posture – see p. 62).

Now let's say one of those muscles is weakened (because of injury or not being trained effectively) – we might notice that our joint sits a little differently and our posture is altered. The joint change is based on whichever muscle is stronger and winning the tug of war.

This is what can happen during pregnancy, as your abdominals stretch and relax to make room for your bump. When the abdominal muscles aren't showing up for their portion of the work in stabilising the trunk, the muscles of the lower back have to turn up and work harder, and they can start to pull your lower spine into extension (because the abdominals are not as good at providing flexion). You may then start to notice that you lean back a little, your lower back becomes more curved and the muscles of the lower back start to get tighter – which doesn't always feel great.

Another common effect of pregnancy is diastasis recti (see p. 167). Defined as a thinning and widening of the linea alba, diastasis recti can occur in anyone, but is often associated with pregnancy. As the bump grows, the rectus abdominis muscles start to move apart, and the linea alba that connects them thins and widens to allow the growth. Studies suggest that up to 100 per cent of women will have some level of diastasis by the time they give birth[18], so this is not something you should panic about. It is thought that it returns to some sort of 'normal' in two thirds of women postnatally. For the remaining third, in whom diastasis persists postnatally, we don't yet know why this is, but core rehabilitation can have a positive effect on performance – and this will be our focus in Part 3.[19]

During pregnancy, your abdominals will continue to lengthen and stretch until labour. Now imagine the sheer change of volume within the abdominal cavity post-birth. The space created by the baby no longer sitting in the uterus is substantial, and many of us are shocked at how long it takes for our tummies to no longer look pregnant. Unlike an elastic band, the abdominals do not simply ping back to their pre-conception length. It takes 9–10 months, perhaps, to get to this length, and it can take a while for them to gradually reduce again. For some women, they may never be the exact same length and strength as pre-conception, but they can definitely improve and remodel.

To do this, however, muscles need stimulation: you need to bring blood to them, you need to challenge them and you need to allow them time to remodel and regain their strength. This too will be a focus in Part 3, where you will learn how to provide just enough stimulation to the core to rebuild its strength without overloading it or slowing your progress.

So the abdominals are arguably the muscles that go through the biggest change during pregnancy, affecting how the body both functions and feels, but there are exercises you can include in your pregnancy training that can help to offset this, support posture and reduce potential tension or pain, as well as others postnatally to speed up recovery. I've got your back on this one, literally, and this book will help you to navigate these incredibly clever adaptations.

The pelvic floor
It's impossible to discuss pregnancy and parenting without mentioning the pelvic floor, so here goes.

The pelvic floor is an area that many of us only consider when an issue arises (like incontinence), yet I would go so far as to say that it is one of the most important parts of the body. Not only does it have some vital functions, but when there are problems with the pelvic floor, they can have a profound effect on your life,

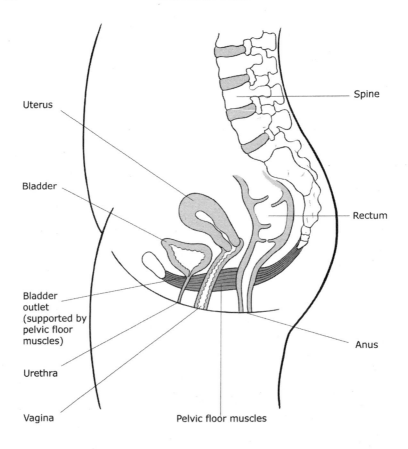

Spine

Uterus

Bladder

Rectum

Bladder outlet (supported by pelvic floor muscles)

Anus

Urethra

Vagina   Pelvic floor muscles

particularly your self-confidence. So let's take a look at what the pelvic floor is.

First, there's the pelvis, the home of the pelvic floor. The pelvis can be imagined as almost a bowl shape, sitting at the top of the legs and the base of the spine. It's formed from two hip bones (the ilia) resembling Mickey Mouse ears. These bones connect at the front to form the pubic symphysis and at the back to join the base of the spine at the sacroiliac joint. Unlike an actual bowl, the pelvis has no base to it, and this is where the pelvic floor comes in handy.

The pelvic floor is made up of layers of muscle tissue that span from the pubic bone at the front of the pelvis, towards the coccyx at the base of the spine, and out towards the sit bones. The pelvic floor forms a hammock of muscles, without which our abdominal contents would essentially fall out of us. The pelvic floor muscles wrap around three holes – the urethra, vagina and anus – and control their constriction and relaxation. As such, the pelvic floor has the following important roles:

- It supports the weight of the pelvic organs, including the bladder, bowel and uterus.
- It controls the passage of urine, faeces and wind.
- It plays a part in sexual function.

The mechanics of the pelvic floor

The pelvic floor is made up of both 'slow-' and 'fast-twitch' muscle fibres. Slow-twitch muscle fibres are endurance muscles (I like to think of them as the long-shift workers) and they are responsible for the main day-to-day functioning of the pelvic floor. The fast-twitch muscle fibres, on the other hand, are the power muscles (or, as I like to imagine them, a back-up army) and they jump into action when there's an emergency (for example, you sneeze and need some extra support); they don't hang around for long – endurance is not their thing – but boy, are they strong!

Both slow- and fast-twitch muscle fibres need to be working well to keep the pelvic floor functioning. The slow-twitch fibres respond best to pelvic floor holds (where you try to contract and hold your pelvic floor for up to 8–10 seconds), and the fast-twitch ones respond best to pelvic floor pulses (fast, short contractions). We'll go into all this in more depth in Part 2, but, hopefully, you now understand why a strong pelvic floor doesn't come from just imagining you're holding in a wee every now and again. The pelvic floor needs specific regular and challenging training to get strong and stay strong. And you'll find everything you need to know about this right here, in these pages.

Now, during pregnancy the uterus grows, as we've seen, and with this growth comes extra weight that pushes down on to the pelvic floor. This, in turn, has to manage the increase in weight and its job gets harder as the pregnancy progresses. This highlights the importance of entering into pregnancy with a pelvic floor that is functional and strong, where possible, to give it the best chance of coping with the extra demands placed on it.

When it comes to labour, during a vaginal birth, the pelvic floor must stretch to allow the baby to pass through the vaginal canal. You'll notice I discuss the concept of 'releasing' the pelvic floor after a pelvic floor contraction later in the book, and this is why: yes, we want a strong pelvic floor that can contract and tighten the vaginal canal, but it also needs to be able to lengthen and stretch for a vaginal birth. Some women may experience trauma/damage to the pelvic floor during labour, but rehabilitation in this area post-labour will make a huge difference for most. I'll discuss this in much more depth in Part 3.

So you can see that pregnancy and labour can put a huge amount of extra strain on the pelvic floor, and because of this some women may notice signs of dysfunction during this time, including the following:

- Urinary or faecal incontinence (the inability to control the passage of urine, faeces or wind, particularly when under increased strain, such as when coughing, sneezing or jumping).
- Pain during intercourse.
- A feeling of heaviness or bulging in the vagina (this can be a sign of a pelvic organ prolapse – POP).

For many, simply practising some pelvic floor exercises (you'll find ones relevant to your stage throughout the book) with good technique will rectify these problems. If in doubt, however, please do ask your GP to refer you to a pelvic health physiotherapist (also known as a fanny magician) – because it may be common, but pelvic floor dysfunction is not 'normal' and does not have to be tolerated.

The glutes

Ok, so I know I said that the core is really important . . . and that the pelvic floor is one of the most important parts of your body . . . but the glutes – well, they are pretty epic, too. I can thank Kim Kardashian in a *very* minor way for helping to remind women to train their glutes, but over the years, I have noticed that the glute muscles are often left behind (no pun intended). Yet they are such an important muscle group for general life and movement, and during pregnancy they really come into their own, offering your growing bump the support it needs as it gets heavier.

The glutes sit at the top of the rear of the legs and wrap around the back and sides of the pelvis. There are three gluteal muscles – gluteus maximus, gluteus medius and gluteus minimus – and together, they play a huge role in movement and stability of the legs and pelvis.

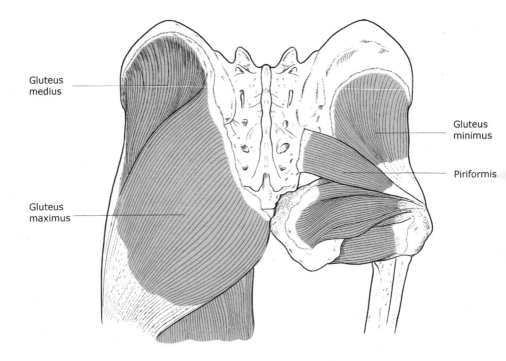

Gluteus medius

Gluteus minimus

Piriformis

Gluteus maximus

Gluteus maximus

Let's start with the most famous of glutes. This, as its name suggests, is the biggest of the glute muscles and it is, in fact, the largest muscle in the whole body. It gives our buttock area the shape we are so familiar with and is the fleshy part we sit on. The gluteus maximus plays a key role in keeping the upper body in an erect position (rather than folding forwards at the hips, such as when sitting) and its main function is to extend the hip (opening the front of the hip and drawing the leg backwards) and externally rotating the thigh (as if you were turning your leg outwards). It also plays a role in stabilising the pelvis and the trunk. You use it when you run, climb stairs, get up from sitting and come out of a hip hinge (you'll get to know hip hinges very well soon).

Gluteus medius

The gluteus medius lies between the gluteus maximus and gluteus minimus and is the primary hip abductor (it takes the leg out to the side). It also plays a role in medial rotation of the thigh (turning your leg inwards) and supports the pelvis when you are on one leg (such as when walking or running), preventing your pelvis from falling sideways.

Gluteus minimus

As its name suggests, this is the smallest of the glute muscles, and it is positioned just beneath the gluteus medius. Its main roles are to stabilise the pelvis (particularly when standing on one leg) and abduct the hip (taking the leg out to the side), but it can also medially rotate the thigh (turning the leg inwards).

Now when the uterus grows and a bump forms, this causes a gradual, but profound increase in weight in the abdominal area, which can have the effect of pulling the pelvis forwards (we call this an anterior tilt). The glutes, however, work together to balance this effect back out, helping to pull the pelvis backwards (we call this a posterior tilt). It's important, therefore, that the glutes are kept active and strong during pregnancy, so that they can achieve this balancing effect. They also help with the stability of the pelvis in movement (walking, running, for example) at a time when more weight is being carried above the pelvis and this skill gets more challenging.

In an ideal world, you would want to go into pregnancy with strong, functional glutes, and then maintain this during pregnancy. Therefore, throughout the book you'll find some great glute activation exercises that I know you'll grow to love.

We've covered a lot in this first part of the book, but now comes the bit where you get to move! Remember, at any point you can come back to this section to get clarity on terminology or to understand more about anatomy in the context of specific exercises. But know that moving your body during pregnancy and postpartum should be fun, enjoyable and feel good, so please don't feel any pressure to do anything that doesn't feel right. You've got this!

Part 2: Your Conception and Pregnancy Workouts

Let's get started

Before we get stuck into your activity plan, there are a few things you should know that will help you to get the most out of it.

Warm-ups and cool-downs

Be honest – how often do you actually warm up before exercising? If you're anything like my new clients over the years, probably not that often (at least, not until they get so bored of me banging on about how important it is). We tend to want to get our trainers on, get our exercise done and then get in the shower. But warm-ups and cool-downs are important, particularly once pregnant, so I would urge you to get into the habit of including them now.

A warm-up is a method of gradually preparing the body for physical activity and is usually a less intense version of what you are about to do. For example, you might walk or jog for a short period as a warm-up for a run. This helps to bring blood to the muscles (which can help with performance and mobility) and potentially reduce your chances of injury. During pregnancy, the body isn't a massive fan of big, rapid changes, so to go from zero activity (sitting on the sofa) to suddenly jumping around your living room for 30 minutes could be a bit of a shock to the system and you might find it makes you light-headed or nauseous. That's why it's important to get into the habit of warming up, rather than just jumping in feet first.

A cool-down is a way of bringing the heart rate back to normal gradually by decreasing the intensity level in stages. Again, when pregnant, you don't want to go from full-on activity to just standing still, as it can cause light-headedness, so a cool-down is a great way to gradually come back to rest.

You'll be using the warm-up and cool-down routines from the first chapter in this part ('Trying to Conceive') throughout your Bump Plan, whenever you're going to be including one or more Sweat exercises in your workout (if you're just throwing a few of the Strength exercises into your day, you don't need to do them, unless you'd like to). The warm-up and cool-down routines will ensure your heart rate is raised – or lowered – gradually.

What is neutral posture?

You'll notice that in many of The Bump Plan exercises you'll be practising over the coming months, the term 'neutral' is used a lot, whether that be neutral posture, neutral pelvis, neutral standing position . . . It's often used in Pilates, too, and it can seem a little confusing at first, so let's get to grips with it here.

For the purposes of this book, I want you to see my use of the word 'neutral' as essentially meaning a sort of middle ground.

The original concept of neutral stems from the idea that our skeletons have an ideal posture that sets our muscles up for success and gives us the least chance of injury. It's thought that lifestyle, genetics and previous injuries can alter our posture out of this 'neutral' position, and we then need to try to bring it back. While this all sounds great, the concept of neutral isn't evidence-based and might not even be possible, so I don't want you to think that you need to have perfect posture, and that if your posture deviates from the concept of neutral at all, you're in some way abnormal or have done something 'wrong'. But the concept of starting certain positions in a more neutral version of your posture can be helpful. And if you know what neutral looks like (in an ideal world), then you know what position to try to aim for in certain moves.

So what *does* neutral posture look like? Let's go back to thinking about it as a sort of middle-ground position, avoiding extremes.

You can see in the diagram on the next page that everything is sort of 'in the middle'. And while it doesn't have to be perfect, and neutral will look different on each of us, based on our own starting postures, it makes for a start position that will usually be a bit more neutral than usual. This can help to set you up for success with each exercise – because if you take a moment to think about your start position and your technique in each move, you might be more likely to activate the correct muscles.

The key, perhaps, is not to overthink it. Moving your body is what's most important, but an awareness of neutral can be really helpful.

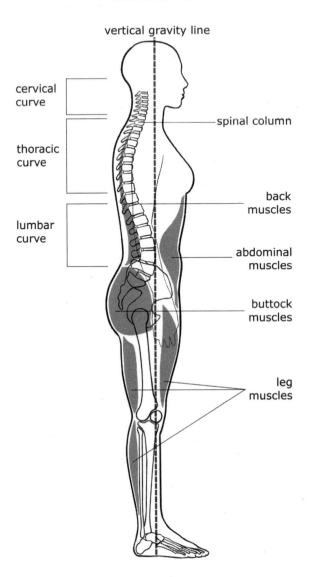

Feet: *roughly hip-width apart and parallel*

Knees: *neither bent nor locked; just a little soft*

Pelvis: *imagine it as a bowl of water you are trying not to spill; neither tucked under nor pushed forwards*

Spine: *a gentle S-shaped curve*

Ribcage: *almost like an upside-down bowl, stacked above the pelvis*

Shoulders: *neither hunched forwards nor aggressively shoved back*

Eyeline: *straight ahead, not looking at the floor or the ceiling*

Make the workouts work for you

All the exercises in this book have been chosen so they can be carried out at home, with no equipment whatsoever; however, a yoga mat or a thick towel would be helpful to stand or lie on if you can source one. And for most exercises I'll be giving you regressions (ways to make them easier) and progressions (ways to make them harder), so you may want to add in a medium resistance band or some light dumbbells in some cases, if that's your jam.

Following your warm-up, we'll move into 'the main-event' exercises: 5x Sweat, 5x Strength. These are designed to be adaptable and there are three main ways you could add them into your life:

1. All of the exercises – both Sweat and Strength – add value to any training you may already be doing, so you could see them as a pick and mix that you can dip into at will and add to your current training plan.
2. Perform the Strength exercises, one after another, for 30–60 seconds each. This is one set. Take a short rest (3–4 minutes) and then you can perform one, two or three more sets, depending on how much time you have available or how challenging it feels for you.
3. Use one of the routine plans I've suggested towards the end of each section.

If you're thinking, 'Hollie, help! I want you to tell me exactly how to plan my workouts,' the table on the next page shows what an example week of routines might look like. You can use this for every chapter in Part 2.

Day 1	Routine: 1 Duration: 60 seconds per exercise Sets: 2 Total minutes: Approx 30
Day 2	Routine: 2 Duration: 60 seconds per exercise Sets: 2 Total minutes: Approx 30
Day 3	Rest day
Day 4	Routine: 1 Duration: 30 seconds per exercise Sets: 4 Total minutes: Approx 30
Day 5	Routine: 2 Duration: 60 seconds per exercise Sets: 1 Total minutes: Approx 20
Day 6	Rest day
Day 7	Routine: 1 Duration: 60 seconds per exercise Sets: 3 Total minutes: Approx 40

You'll also notice that for each exercise I state at what stage of your journey it is safe to perform it, for example, *TTC, pregnancy weeks 0–6 and 7–12, and postnatal phase 2*. This is so that you can continue to use exercises you have learnt (and loved) in previous sections, throughout your parenting journey. My hope is that you start to really know your body, what it needs, what it enjoys, and start to build up a bank of exercises you really love to include in your weekly movement!

Where I state *'entire pregnancy, if comfortable'* this means that you can continue with this exercise during pregnancy, if it feels good, you are managing your core pressure well (see p. 174), there is no aggressive hard-doming (see p. 169), and your pelvic floor is coping. You may find you are able to complete said exercise until 40 weeks, or it may mean you can complete it until 12 weeks – just listen to your body and stop when it no longer feels right for you.

Pelvic floor exercises

Throughout Parts 2 and 3 of this book, you'll notice that I give you lots of pelvic floor exercises and visualisations to test out and practise. Now really, these are to help you nail your pelvic floor workout technique, not full workouts in themselves. This is because your pelvic floor workout will always be the same and is based on the current guidance from the NHS, as follows:

- 10 × slow holds – where you activate your pelvic floor (squeeze and lift) and try to hold for up to 10 seconds
- 10 × fast pulses – where you activate your pelvic floor (squeeze and lift) rapidly and then release immediately

This combination of slow and fast contractions should be practised 3–4 times per day (yes, I know it seems a lot) and takes time to work. It's important that the workout feels challenging (this will encourage strength gains) and that you persevere with it. I promise it'll be worth it.

To really get the most out of your time spent training your pelvic floor, as above, it's important to have good technique and an awareness of where the pelvic floor is and how it functions (see pp. 51–55). The exercises and visualisations in this book will help you to work your pelvic floor like an absolute boss, building it to be stronger and more functional. Practise them alongside your pelvic floor workout to really make the most of your efforts.

It should be noted that some women will not necessarily benefit from traditional pelvic floor exercises. For example, those who have been diagnosed with a hypertonic pelvic floor (where it is in a constant state of contraction or spasm) should avoid the workout described above, and instead request advice and support from their GP or pelvic health physiotherapist (AKA magician) to help them relax and release their pelvic floor.

Right, that's all the admin done. Now let's get started...

TTC – trying to conceive

~~~~~~

If you've picked up this book already pregnant, you can skip this chapter and head straight to p. 96, but if you've decided to start – or grow – a family, or maybe you're already trying to conceive (TTC), this is for you. What an exciting, potentially anxious and slightly unpredictable time this is.

Staying active while TTC – why it's so important

We all come to the TTC journey with different backgrounds, fertility journeys, previous pregnancy experiences and more, so it's important to keep in mind that we'll all also have different hopes, dreams and emotions. I mention this because I often see the TTC period being sugar-coated and spoken about in terms of 'excitement', 'fun' and 'lots of shagging', but for some people this may not be their experience, and it's important we consider *all* journeys.

For me, this was the time where I really 'needed' exercise. I leaned heavily on it to support my mental health and mood while navigating TTC and found it to be an anchor. While TTC for my second baby, I also had the hindsight of knowing just how demanding pregnancy can be, and I really wanted to enter my next pregnancy feeling strong, capable and with a seriously functional pelvic floor (first time around, I struggled with urinary stress incontinence, where you leak urine when sneezing/coughing/jumping).

I believe it's important that we see physical activity as a vital part of TTC. There are so many incredible, proven, health benefits to staying active through all stages of life, and by doing so while TTC, you are giving yourself the best chance of actually conceiving and then experiencing a comfortable, healthy pregnancy. So let's do this!

What do I need to know?

Now I mentioned in Part 1 that official physical activity guidelines are scarce at present when it comes to those who are TTC. This is partly because this isn't considered a distinct group of individuals at present when it comes to physical activity; plus, there's the fact that at some point while TTC, women may be pregnant without realising, and so straddle two groups.

So when TTC, you can either put yourself into the 'general adult population' category (and use the guidelines listed on p. 12) or the 'pregnant population' category (and use the guidelines listed on p. 24). To be honest, they are similar, the main difference being the intensity of the cardiovascular activity (moderate intensity is advised during pregnancy, while the general adult population can work at a moderate, vigorous or very vigorous intensity).

With this is mind, it's also worth considering where you are on your TTC journey. If, say, you are simply flirting with the idea but haven't actively started trying, you might want to stick to the general adult population guidelines for now. If, on the other hand, you are at the point where you're hoping each month for those two blue lines, you might feel more comfortable with the pregnancy guidelines. It's really a case of whatever feels right for you. So let's just remind ourselves of those two sets of guidelines.

The CMOs' physical activity guidelines for adults[1]:

- **Include strengthening activity.** Adults need to include activity that strengthens their musculoskeletal system at least twice per week. This should involve the major muscle groups of the upper and lower body and could take the form of weightlifting at the gym, carrying heavy shopping or activities such as racquet sports or Pilates. The aim here is to improve muscle function, bone health and balance.
- **Include cardiovascular activity.** Each week adults should aim for at least 150 minutes of moderate intensity or 75 minutes of vigorous intensity activity or even shorter durations of very vigorous activity, or a mixture of all the above.
- **Reduce sedentary time.** Adults should aim to minimise the amount of time spent sedentary, and where possible break up long periods of inactivity with at least light physical activity.

And the CMOs' physical activity guidelines for pregnant women[2]:

Healthy pregnant women, experiencing an uncomplicated pregnancy, should aim to accumulate at least 150 minutes of moderate intensity physical activity per week, and include muscle strengthening activities twice a week.

Throughout this book, you'll be given exercise ideas to boost both your cardiovascular and musculoskeletal strength at specific stages. As mentioned earlier, these are split into Strength exercises to target your musculoskeletal strength and Sweat exercises to target your cardiovascular strength. I'll give you a breakdown of how you can use them to create a 'workout' for yourself but it's also worth remembering that *all* activity counts towards the physical activity guidelines. That walk to the train station in the morning? It counts. The deep clean of the bathroom before your family come to visit? That counts. And the sex you're potentially having? That counts, too.

What are we focusing on at this stage?

While we are trying to meet the official physical activity guidelines, and all activity counts, I'd be lying if I didn't admit – as a complete posture and functional movement nerd – that there are some specifics I want to really focus on. I talked a lot in Part 1 about the changes our bodies go through when pregnant, and how these changes can challenge us. I therefore think it's worth thinking of pregnancy as an upcoming marathon. It's a long one (9–10 months is one hell of an endurance race), and it's ever-changing, too (what challenges you at 12 weeks will be different at 36 weeks).

With that in mind, it's wise to consider the TTC stage as pre-race. You wouldn't enter a marathon with no training beforehand (I once did a half marathon without training and it was horrific); rather, you want to use this time to really think about what your body requires from you for pregnancy, and work on that now.

Given that babies grow in the abdominal cavity, and the abdominals will stretch to make room for a growing uterus, it really helps to go into pregnancy with a strong, functional core that works effectively. This will help to provide support to the spine as your bump grows and could also help in speeding up postnatal recovery. While TTC, there are no limitations on the core work you can do (other than your own ability), so it's also the perfect time to get those abdominal exercises in, before the logistics of having a bump come into play.

A strong, functional pelvic floor is also important. I mentioned that I suffered with urinary stress incontinence when pregnant with my first child, Freya. This was because I hadn't prioritised my own pelvic floor training. I spoke all day about the pelvic floor but didn't lead by example. If you can go into pregnancy with a pelvic floor that is working well, you'll be less likely to suffer with pelvic floor dysfunction as the demand placed on it grows (due to the expanding uterus).

You also need to think about good cardiovascular fitness. During pregnancy, up to 50 per cent more blood is gained in the body. That blood has to be pumped around the body (including to the placenta) by the cardiovascular system. So get your cardiovascular strength up now, and then you can focus on maintaining it through pregnancy.

Your exercises: TTC

So now, without further ado, let's get started on your physical activity programme.

Warm-up exercises

You will be referring back to these warm-up exercises through-out the plan.

Perform each of the following for 30–60 seconds.

Marching/walking on the spot

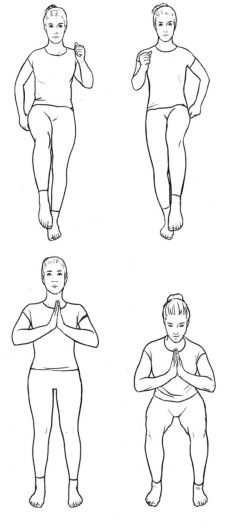

A nice, easy one to start with. Begin marching on the spot, starting with slow, low legs, and swinging your arms, building up the speed and the height of your legs gradually. Aim to get some ankle mobility in here, too, by exaggerating flexing and pointing your ankle as you march.

Squats

Stand with your feet either hip-width apart and in a parallel position or in a 'sumo squat' position (feet wider than hip-width apart and knees and feet turned out). As you inhale, bend the knees, hinge forwards slightly and sit your bottom down, as though you're trying to sit on a chair. Aim to keep your spine neutral as you do this. As you exhale, push through your feet to bring yourself back to your start position.

Skater stretches

Stand with your feet parallel and as wide as is comfortable for your pelvis, your hands in prayer position at your chest. Bend your left knee and drop your hips as low as is comfortable, feeling a stretch along the inside of your right leg. Push through your left leg to

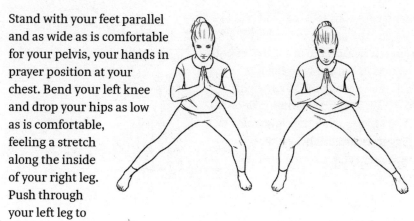

come back to the start position before repeating on the other side. Aim to press through the bent knee to come back to your start position, rather than pulling yourself up with your straight leg.

Shoulder circles

Stand with your hands on your shoulders and elbows out to the sides. Rocking from side to side (to prevent you cooling down), draw circles with your elbows, opening up the chest and loosening off the shoulders. After 30 seconds, change direction.

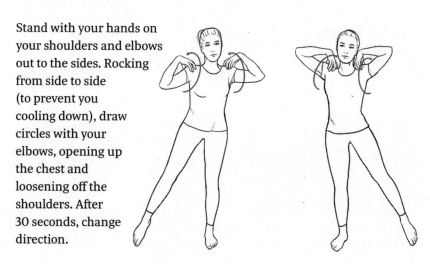

Calf peddling

Stand with your feet hip-width apart.
Keeping the pelvis relatively still, lift
your left heel off the ground keeping
the toes in contact with the floor
(calf raise), while the whole right
foot stays in contact with the floor.
Then swap, so that the right ankle is
in a calf raise and the left foot
remains in contact with the floor.
Repeat.

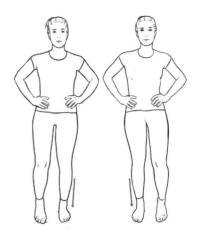

Ankle circles

Standing, shift your weight to your left leg. Rotate your right ankle in
a circle one way 3–5 times, then reverse it, before repeating on the
other side.

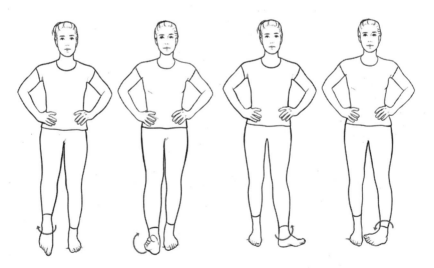

Now you've completed your warm-up, let's move on to the
Strength and Sweat exercises.

Strength exercises

The following are designed to give you the muscle strengthening activity you need to meet the guidelines we've discussed.

Abdominal hollowing (suitable for TTC, entire pregnancy, if comfortable, and postnatal all phases)

This is a great exercise for teaching you how to activate your core and boost stability in the pelvis and lower back. It strengthens the pelvic floor and transversus abdominis muscle which wraps around your trunk like a corset.

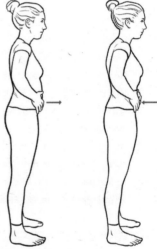

1. Stand in a neutral position, with your hands resting on your tummy near your belly button.
2. Inhale, and then, as you exhale, think about lifting up your pelvic floor and activating your transversus abdominis.
3. As you inhale, relax.
4. Repeat.

TIP: There are a few ways you can visualise activating your transversus abdominis: you could imagine that you are drawing in your tummy slightly, that someone is tightening up a corset around your waist or that you are trying to do up a pair of tight jeans. What you should feel under your hands is a slight pulling inwards of your tummy. It's not aggressive, and you should still be able to breathe.

REGRESSION: start with just the pelvic floor lift in step 2, or just the transversus abdominis activation, then build up to doing them both together.

PROGRESSION: add a 10-second hold in at the end but ensure you can still breathe or talk while holding.

Ab prep (suitable for TTC and pregnancy weeks 0–6 and 7–12)

This exercise is a great way to stimulate the rectus abdominis and obliques. Performed correctly, it can also teach you how to stabilise the pelvis and lower back during movement. A simple, but effective abdominal exercise.

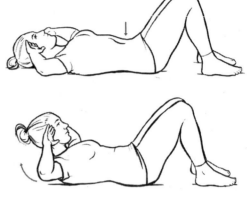

1. Start lying on your back, knees bent, with your feet roughly hip-width apart and parallel.
2. Bring your fingers to your temples, elbows wide.
3. Inhale and nod your head slightly, as though giving yourself a little double chin.
4. As you exhale, start to lift the head and shoulders away from the floor, flexing your upper spine, and drawing your ribcage down towards your hip bones.
5. Inhale to stay here, and exhale to lower back down with control.

TIP: While performing this move, try not to dig your lower back (your lumbar spine) into the floor, or aggressively press into your feet. You should be using your abdominals to pull you up, rather than the floor to push you up.

REGRESSION: if you find your neck aches in this move, you could interlace your fingers and use your hands behind your head, almost like a hammock to support it on the lift. You could also exhale to lift the head and shoulders, and inhale to lower them, rather than including the hold.

PROGRESSION: you could add weight by straightening your arms above your head (almost like you are diving). You could also do this with your legs in tabletop (lifting your feet, so your knees are at right angles and your lower legs are parallel to the floor), rather than with your feet on the floor.

Glute kickbacks (suitable for TTC, entire pregnancy, if comfortable, and postnatal phases 1 and 2)

This is one of my favourite exercises for activating the glute and hamstring muscles, while also encouraging core stability. The glutes and hamstrings will provide support for the pelvis in future pregnancies.

1. Start on hands and knees, with a neutral spine, knees hip-width apart and your core slightly engaged. You can do this by engaging both your pelvic floor and your transversus abdominis lightly, so it feels like a corset is tightening around your waist.
2. Bend your right knee and imagine there is a tennis ball behind it that you don't want to drop.
3. Keeping your spine neutral, start to lift the right leg up away from the floor, bringing your foot towards the ceiling.
4. Inhale to lower it back to the floor.
5. Repeat as required, and then switch legs.

TIP: The aim here is to use your glute muscles to extend the hip and pull the leg up towards the ceiling, not your lower back. Therefore, your pelvis and spine should be staying still, as the leg lifts and lowers. Remember ... don't lose the tennis ball behind the knee; it gives the hamstring something to do! Also, try not to lean to the side too much as you do this – it will require some core strength.

REGRESSION: if you find this position uncomfortable, you could come down on to your forearms, rather than weight bearing on your hands. You could start with small lifts at first and gradually increase as you feel more stable.

PROGRESSION: rather than an imaginary tennis ball behind the knee, you could put a real dumbbell there to add resistance. You could also add a 10-second hold or 10 seconds of pulses at the end of your set.

Hip hinges (suitable for TTC, entire pregnancy, if comfortable, and postnatal phases 1 and 2)

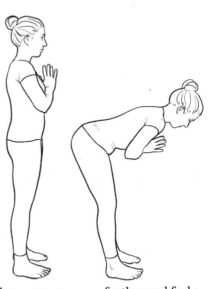

A hip hinge is a fundamental exercise to learn. Many others involve a hip hinge (squats and lunges, for example) and we also use them often during the day (bending over to turn on the bath, look into cots, wipe kids' noses, etc.) so it's worth getting good at them.

1. Start in a neutral standing position, with your hands in prayer position at your chest.
2. On your next inhale, start to hinge at your hips, looking as though you are bowing. Eventually, you'll hit a point where you can go no further and feel a stretch up the back of the legs.
3. Exhale to press the feet into the floor and bring yourself back to your start position.

TIP: We are aiming for a hip hinge here, which means that the only joint to really change is the hip joint. So the knees stay soft, but do not bend (it's not a squat) and the back stays in a neutral position. Try to use the backs of the legs to pull yourself back up to standing, rather than simply leaning back. If you experience lower back tension here, try activating your core a little more for extra lumbar support.

REGRESSION: start with a small range of movement, rather than hitting your end point. You could also start the exercise standing a few centimetres away from a wall and, as you hinge forwards, bring your bottom backwards to the wall for support.

PROGRESSION: try adding extra resistance by holding dumbbells, a kettlebell or barbell, or by standing on a resistance band holding the ends in your hands.

Aeroplanes (suitable for TTC, entire pregnancy, if comfortable, and postnatal phase 2)

Performed correctly, this is a really spicy exercise! It's a great way to target the gluteus medius and gluteus minimis and encourage pelvic stability. It may take some practice, though.

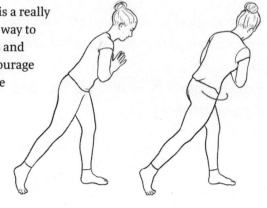

1. Start in a neutral standing position.
2. Hip hinge to halfway, bringing yourself out to about 45°, if you can.
3. Shift your weight over to your left leg and put your right foot behind you on the floor (so you are in a staggered stance).
4. Inhale and start to rotate your pelvis to the left, as far as it will go.
5. As you exhale, push your left foot into the floor and rotate your pelvis back to face forwards.
6. Repeat as required, then switch legs.

TIP: Imagine you have headlights on your hip bones. When your hips point forwards your headlights should shine on to your mat, and when you rotate, imagine the lights shining off the side of your mat. This is about the pelvis rotating on top of the leg, but you may find your standing leg tries to bend – that's cheating!

REGRESSION: you could try the initial technique without the hip hinge, as the further forwards you hinge, the harder the exercise becomes.

PROGRESSION: you could lift your back leg off the floor and have it hovering in the air, so that you lose that base of support.

Sweat exercises

These are designed to help you meet the cardiovascular exercise requirement in the CMOs' guidelines we've talked about.

Half-burpees (suitable for TTC and entire pregnancy, if comfortable)

This exercise really challenges your shoulder strength and endurance, but also your core strength. It should be quite an explosive exercise, but technique is also very important.

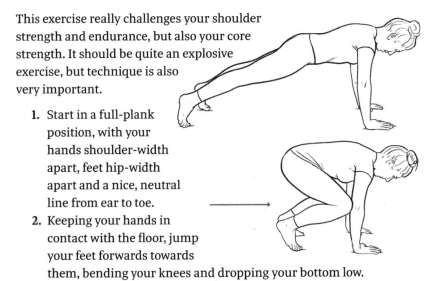

1. Start in a full-plank position, with your hands shoulder-width apart, feet hip-width apart and a nice, neutral line from ear to toe.
2. Keeping your hands in contact with the floor, jump your feet forwards towards them, bending your knees and dropping your bottom low.
3. Jump back out into your plank position.
4. Repeat.

TIP: Be careful of allowing the hips to fall too low when in your plank – it would be preferable for them to be too high rather than too low. And try to put the weight through your arms when jumping, so that you are better supported on landing and do so as gently as possible.

REGRESSION: rather than jumping in and out, you could step one foot at a time in and out to your plank position. This will also reduce the impact on your joints.

PROGRESSION: you could pick up the pace or turn this into a full burpee – simply jump up to standing after jumping the feet to the hands, and then drop back down and jump back out to a plank.

Plyometric lunges (suitable for TTC and entire pregnancy, if comfortable)

This is a great cardiovascular exercise that challenges your strength, endurance and stability. It may feel quite wobbly at first, so take your time.

1. Start in a standing position and step your right foot forwards, so that you are in a staggered stance.
2. Bend both knees, lean forwards slightly, and you'll be in a lunge position.
3. Now jump up and swap the legs over, so you land in the same lunge position but with the left leg in front.
4. Repeat.

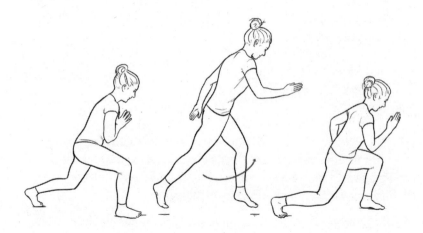

TIP: This can get tiring very quickly, so do slow down if/when you need to. Try to land as softly as you can, and feel free to use your arms to help you jump up and give you some momentum.

REGRESSION: instead of jumping up and switching the legs over, simply step the front leg back in and then lunge forwards with the other leg. You can also reduce the range of movement by not stepping as far forwards or bending your knees as deeply.

PROGRESSION: you could pick up the pace; or try to land as quietly as possible (this is much harder).

Shoulder taps (suitable for TTC, entire pregnancy, if comfortable, and postnatal phase 2)

This is a great way to challenge your core and shoulder stability, while giving you the option of which type of plank works best for you.

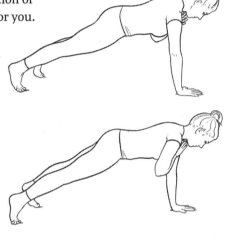

1. Start in either a half- or full-plank position, with hands shoulder-width apart and a nice, neutral line from ear to toe.
2. Lift your left hand away from the floor and tap your right shoulder with it.
3. Replace your left hand, then take the right hand away from the floor and tap your left shoulder.
4. Repeat.

TIP: The challenge here is stability – trying not to rock from side to side when performing this exercise. Think about pressing down through the supporting arm (the one in contact with the floor) and keep the hips facing downwards (not rotating as you move).

REGRESSION: try this in four-point kneeling (hands and knees) first, and slow it right down, before building up to a half-plank position.

PROGRESSION: you could hold dumbbells in your hands and bring them with you as you reach towards your opposite shoulder.

Commandos (suitable for TTC, entire pregnancy, if comfortable, and postnatal phase 2)

I always feel strong and powerful when I do this exercise – mainly because of its name. It's a great one for building strength in the triceps, pectorals and core.

1. Start in either a half- or full-plank position, with hands shoulder-width apart and a nice, neutral line from ear to toe.
2. Lower yourself down on to your left forearm, and then your right forearm (so you are now resting on both of them).
3. Use your left hand to push yourself up, followed by the right one, to return to your start position.
4. Repeat.

TIP: Try to alternate the arm that moves first each time – so you might go left forearm, right forearm, left hand, right hand; then right forearm, left forearm, right hand, left hand. And try to keep the pelvis as still as you can as you move (so not too much rotating from side to side).

REGRESSION: try this in four-point kneeling (hands and knees) first, and slow it right down, before building up to a half-plank position.

PROGRESSION: increase the pace; or use the hardest full-plank option.

Full floor to ceilings (suitable for TTC, entire pregnancy, if comfortable, and postnatal phase 2)

This exercise mimics bending down and picking something up off the floor and is therefore incredibly functional and useful for everyday life!

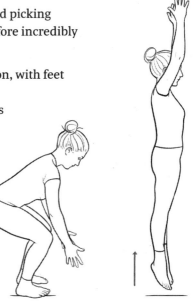

1. Start in a neutral standing position, with feet hip-width apart.
2. Squat down and reach your hands down in front of you, almost as if you are picking up a box from the floor.
3. Push through your feet and jump up into the air, as if you are trying to touch the ceiling.
4. Repeat.

TIP: This exercise should be explosive – but do try to land as softly as you can, aiming to keep the spine as neutral as possible as you move (rather than hunching over to reach the floor, for example).

REGRESSION: slow the whole move down; or remove the jump at the top and simply come back to standing in neutral each time.

PROGRESSION: pick up the pace, or hold dumbbells in your hands to add resistance.

Cool-down exercises

You will be referring back to these cool-down exercises throughout the plan.
Perform each of these for 30–60 seconds.

Marching on the spot

Just as you did in the warm-up,
begin marching on the spot,
starting with high, fast legs and
swinging your arms, reducing
the speed and the height of your
legs gradually, until your
marching is at a walking pace.

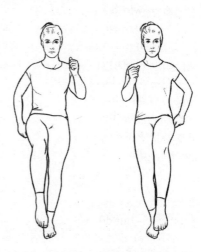

Skater stretches

Stand with your feet parallel and as far apart as is comfortable for your
pelvis, and your hands in prayer position at your chest. Bend your left knee
and drop your hips as low as is comfortable, feeling a stretch along the
inside of your right leg and hold for 5 seconds (the hold is what makes this
exercise slightly different from the version you did in the warm-up). Push
through your left leg to come back to the start position before repeating on
the other side. Aim to press through the bent knee to come back to your
start position, rather than pulling yourself up with your straight leg.

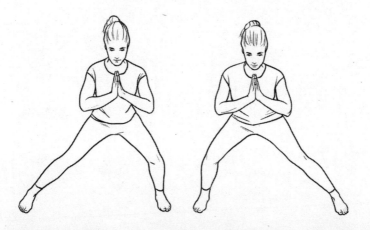

Arm circles

These are similar to the shoulder circles in the warm-up (see p. 75).
Stand with your arms straight out to the sides. Slowly rocking from foot to
foot, draw circles with your arms. Change direction at the halfway point.

Calf peddling

Stand with your feet hip-width apart. Keeping the pelvis relatively
still, lift your right heel off the ground, keeping the toes in contact with
the floor (calf raise) while the left foot
stays in contact with the floor. Swap, so
that the left ankle is in a calf raise and
the right foot stays in contact with the
floor. Repeat.

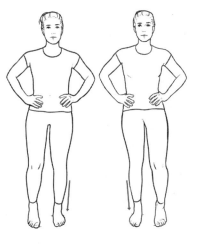

Ankle circles

Stand and shift your weight to your left
leg. Rotate your right ankle in a circle
one way 3–5 times, then reverse, before
repeating on the other side.

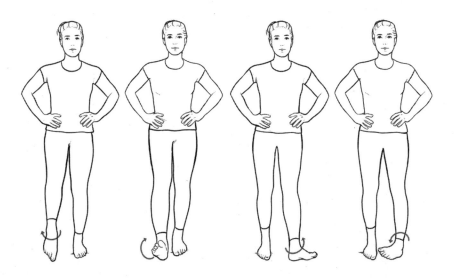

Example routines

Below, you'll find two example routines. Routine 1 combines all of the exercise options. Routine 2 combines all of the Sweat exercises with a rest period (which you do not have to utilise). Feel free to repeat the routines to help you build up to the recommended 150 minutes of physical activity per week (an example week could be 5 x 30 minute workouts).

Routine 1

- *Warm-up*
- Plyometric lunges: 30–60 seconds
- Abdominal hollowing: 30–60 seconds
- Half-burpees: 30–60 seconds
- Ab prep: 30–60 seconds
- Shoulder taps: 30–60 seconds
- Glute kickbacks: 30–60 seconds
- Commandos: 30–60 seconds
- Hip hinges: 30–60 seconds
- Full floor to ceilings: 30–60 seconds
- Aeroplanes: 30-60 seconds
- *Repeat or cool-down* (if repeating, don't exceed four sets and be sure to include a rest period if you need it between sets)

Routine 2

- *Warm-up*
- Half-burpees: 30–60 seconds
- Rest – marching on the spot: 60 seconds
- Plyometric lunges: 30–60 seconds
- Rest – marching on the spot: 60 seconds
- Shoulder taps: 30–60 seconds

- Rest – marching on the spot: 60 seconds
- Commandos: 30–60 seconds
- Rest – marching on the spot: 60 seconds
- Full floor to ceilings: 30–60 seconds
- *Repeat or cool-down* (if repeating, don't exceed four sets and be sure to include a rest period if you need it between sets)

Your pelvic floor exercise

We discussed the importance and role of the pelvic floor in Part 1 (see pp. 51–55) and how vital it is that this area is as strong and as functional as possible when entering pregnancy. Pregnancy puts a huge amount of strain on the pelvic floor, and prevention of pelvic floor dysfunction is better than cure.

I can vouch for the fact that it takes work, though. A couple of pelvic floor squeezes while you are waiting at the traffic lights won't quite cut it. You need to treat the pelvic floor like any other muscle in the body – it has to be trained properly, regularly, until it tires. So as we go along, at this point in every chapter I'll be sharing pelvic floor exercises, techniques and visualisations that will help you to really understand how to train this area for success.

Let's start with the basics with the pelvic floor finder.

Pelvic floor finder

We are often told that to activate the pelvic floor we need to simply imagine holding in a wee – but this really isn't a good enough cue and tends to favour the front section of the pelvic floor only.

Instead, you need to really get a feel for where the pelvic floor is, and how to activate *all* of it. In Part 1, we discussed the anatomy of the pelvic floor, and how it spans the base of the pelvis and is actually bigger than many people realise, so feel free to refer back to this on p. 52 if you need to remind yourself.

This particular exercise will help you to get more bang for your buck from your pelvic floor holds and pulses. It'll also help you to get a feel for engaging the entire pelvic floor musculature, and you can use this technique when you do your pelvic floor workout.

1. Start in a comfortable position – this might be seated, lying, side-lying, standing.
2. Close your eyes (this will help you to focus internally) and try to clear your mind.
3. Focus on your breathing by bringing your awareness to breathing in and out through your nose. Relax your jaw and ensure your tongue is relaxed in your mouth.
4. Try to picture the three holes that the pelvic floor wraps around (the urethra, the vaginal opening and the anus).
5. Focusing first on the urethra, take a big breath in and, as you exhale, think about closing and lifting it, as you would if you were trying to hold in a wee or stop one mid-flow.
6. Inhale to release and relax; exhale to repeat.
7. Repeat 5 times and then rest for a moment.
8. Now focusing on the vaginal opening, take a big inhale and, as you exhale, imagine squeezing and lifting the vaginal opening. (Some people find it helpful to imagine gripping something with the vagina – for example, a finger/penis/sex toy; or you might prefer thinking of squeezing the labia towards each other.)
9. Inhale to release and relax; exhale to repeat.
10. Repeat 5 times and then rest for a moment.
11. Finally, focusing on the anus, take a big inhale and, as you exhale, imagine squeezing and lifting the anus, as if you were trying to hold in wind or a poo, or stopping a poo midway.
12. Inhale to release and relax; exhale to repeat.
13. Repeat 5 times and then rest for a moment.
14. Now bring it all together: inhale and, as you exhale, squeeze and lift all three holes, combining everything you have practised.
15. Inhale to release; exhale to repeat.
16. Repeat 5 times and then rest.

TIP: Hopefully, visualising all three holes in this exercise really helps you to increase your pelvic floor engagement and activate more of the pelvic floor musculature. You want to achieve a sense of the entire pelvic floor activating and lifting. If you find that one of the holes/areas seems harder to engage than the others, you could spend more time focusing on it until its strength improves.

I'm going through IVF, can I still stay active?

By Stacey Draper, university researcher and PhD candidate

According to NICE,[3] an estimated one in seven couples in the UK are affected by infertility and the UK fertility regulator (HFEA) say around 91 per cent of people seeking fertility treatment are heterosexual partnerships and the remainder are those in same-sex relationships, single women, and those using surrogacy.[4] Demand for fertility treatment is rising, so improving fertility treatment outcomes has become a topic of interest for healthcare professionals and those trying to conceive.

As we know, physical activity has many benefits such as reduced risks of cardiovascular disease, cancers, diabetes and enhanced psychological wellbeing.[5] However, the effect of physical activity on fertility treatment outcomes is controversial within the current research and practice, so it can be confusing for those undergoing fertility treatment to know what to do. Particularly as this unique period of time comes with a lot of emotional, physical, and psychological difficulties, not least the intense desire for a successful outcome. Despite evidence to suggest fertility treatment outcomes can be influenced by physical activity levels, there is currently very little evidence-based guidance available to women in the UK who are undergoing fertility treatment.

What does the research say?

Research shows that physical activity can affect fertility and fertility treatment outcomes, although findings are varied and inconsistent. Most studies found that women who participate in moderate level physical activity demonstrate improved fertility treatment outcomes[3] whereas those who engage in vigorous intensities and higher frequencies of physical activity have shown increased rates of subfertility, infertility and delayed time to spontaneous pregnancy.[6, 7] These findings suggest exercise intensity and frequency can impact fertility treatment outcomes. However, it's important to note that many of the studies published rely on self-reporting physical activity, intensity, weight loss and dietary habits.

While there is evidence to support the safety of being active for the majority of women, research shows that women are still worried about physical activity or even commit to complete bed rest during this time.[8, 9, 10] Concerns about being active during treatment cycles often stem from outdated research that recommended bed rest following procedures.[11] Research has since suggested there are no benefits of bed rest on IVF treatment outcomes and can even be detrimental. This is thought to be due to negative psychological symptoms, such as stress, anxiety, and depression.[12]

Intensity, types and frequency of physical activity can have varied effects on fertility treatment outcomes. For example, one study found that only greater time spent engaging in specific activities (aerobics, rowing, ski or stair machine) was associated with a higher probability of live birth. These results were for women who engaged in 1.5 hours or more per week, compared to women who engaged in 0 hours per week of the same activities. Another study looked at grouping women into a low activity group or a moderate activity group and found that the moderate activity led to an increased implantation rate and live birth rate. On further investigation, a positive correlation was found between live birth results and energy expenditure, and physical activity levels during treatment but not prior to treatment. This suggests that timing may be important and being physically active during fertility treatments is more likely to positively affect treatment outcomes.

However, despite evidence supporting physical activity during fertility treatment, some studies have found the opposite to be true. Research demonstrates that women who are engaging in high levels of vigorous intensity physical activity are more likely to be diagnosed with infertility. A large study of 2,323 couples undergoing their first IVF cycle found that women who were physically active for more than 4 hours per week for 1-9 years were 40 per cent less likely to have a successful live birth than those who were not regularly active.[13, 14] Additionally, these women were almost three times more likely to experience cycle cancellation and twice as likely to experience implantation failure or pregnancy loss than those who did not report regular physical activity. Another study compared women from the highest physical activity group to the lowest and found the highest group were more commonly diagnosed with an ovulation disorder or diminished ovarian reserve.[15] This aligns with previous research which suggests doing a lot of intense activity is associated with an irregular menstrual cycle, and is therefore most commonly seen in athletes.

All of this is confusing, but what the research shows is that it's the intensity and frequency of physical activity that influences treatment outcomes. Most studies found no adverse effects on treatment outcomes on women who are physically active and therefore, it's recommended that you do some light to moderate daily activity throughout treatment.

Pregnancy weeks 0–6

I understand that at this stage not that many women will know for sure that they are pregnant. By the time an off-the-shelf pregnancy test can confirm a pregnancy it is usually already around 4 weeks in, but for those who are actively TTC, suffer with fertility issues or are navigating IVF, I'm sure you're taking those tests frequently and will know as soon as is possible. So huge congratulations, to those of you who are here. I hope you're feeling positive and have lots of support around you.

In Part 1, we took a deep dive into why staying active during pregnancy is so important. The proven physical and mental health benefits are vast, and there really is so much you can do safely. I know this stage might feel daunting – particularly if this is your first pregnancy, this has been a long journey, or you've suffered a previous loss – but in the coming pages, I'll guide you through what to do and how.

Your body

It's unlikely that you'll be experiencing any pregnancy-related physical symptoms yet, which means that you'll hopefully have enough energy currently to meet your physical activity guidelines (you can revisit these on p. 24). I say this with a caveat, however – because not everyone will have been active pre-conception, whether due to fertility treatment, illness, lack of childcare or nervousness around overdoing it. Or maybe you just don't really *love* exercise yet and you're hoping that this book will help you to find your mojo now you're pregnant. (It will!)

What you need to know

If you weren't active before conception, now is the time to start (although it's worth familiarising yourself with the contraindications information on p. 30 first). There are so many proven benefits, and it really isn't rocket science (although it can feel like it at times). I would just advise that you ease yourself in, starting with shorter workouts, and gradually build up as you feel comfortable.

If you were already active before pregnancy, I want you to try to maintain your fitness levels. For some of you, your workouts might look slightly different during pregnancy (contact sports, diving and skydiving are not advised), but it needn't feel boring or uninspiring. You can still get your heart rate up, your cheeks flushed, your body moving and generally enjoy physical activity as before. Just make sure you've swotted up on the information in Part 1 around the current physical activity guidelines from the wonderful UK CMOs (see p. 24).

What is the focus in weeks 0–6?

The current guidelines from the UK CMOs are that we train at a moderate intensity during pregnancy, so this is a great time to get used to this concept. It is explained in greater detail on p. 16, but essentially, it means still being able to talk, but not sing, while exercising.

For example, let's say you're a regular runner, and you usually complete a 5k run once a week. I'd love you to continue with that for as long as you feel comfortable doing so, but just check while running that you could still hold a conversation. On your next run, pretend you are telling someone about your weekend plans, or where you went on your last holiday. If you can talk, you're all good; if not, slow it down so that you can. Over the next 9 months you'll more than likely find that your 5k run time will need to be much longer, as you'll have to run slower to stay at a moderate level. Or maybe it will end up being a 3k run or a 5k walk instead. That is all good – just keep moving at that moderate level.

Regarding your Bump Plan Strength exercises, you'll see that they're pretty core dominant. Yes, you're pregnant, but you won't have a bump yet that affects the core work you need to be doing. So make the most of this time, and include exercises that just won't be possible or comfortable further down the line. This way, you'll create a strong, functional core ahead of a bump showing up.

With your Sweat exercises, you can practise your moderate intensity 'talk test' and play around with the regressions and progressions listed to see what works best for you right now.

Your exercises: weeks 0–6

Your warm-up and cool-down exercises can be found on pp. 74–76 and 87–88. Now let's get moving! Here are your 'Strength' and 'Sweat' exercises for this first part of your pregnancy.

Strength exercises

Criss-crosses (suitable for TTC, pregnancy weeks 0–6 and 7–12 and postnatal phase 2)

A great rotation exercise for strengthening the rectus abdominis and obliques, plus most of us don't get enough spine rotation in our daily lives.

1. Start by lying on your back, legs in a tabletop position, fingers to temples and elbows wide.
2. Lift your head and shoulders gently away from the mat, so your upper back is flexed.
3. Inhale, and then, as you exhale, extend your left leg out, as low as you can keep your pelvis neutral and rotate your upper body towards the right knee (which is still in tabletop).
4. Inhale as you come back through the centre, and then exhale as you extend the right leg and rotate towards the left knee.
5. Repeat.

TIP: This is about rotating the ribcage towards the opposite knee, not just the elbow. Often, I see people whose spines stay in the centre, but their arms are moving all over the place. Instead, think opposite rib to opposite hip (rather than opposite elbow to opposite knee).

REGRESSION: keep your feet on the floor, instead of up in tabletop. This will remove some challenge from the hip flexors and reduce the load of the core. If you struggle with neck ache here, you could interlace the fingers and support your head in your hands while in flexion.

PROGRESSION: try taking the extended leg a little lower (closer to the mat), so that you have to work harder to maintain a neutral pelvis. You could add in a 10-second hold on each side at the end, or 10 seconds of pulses on each side to finish.

Half-roll backs (suitable for TTC, pregnancy weeks 0–6, 7–12 and 13–19, and postnatal phase 2)

This exercise challenges your core strength, hip flexor control and also encourages some lumbar flexion, which can help to release a tight lower back.

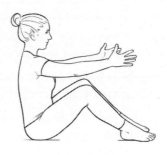

1. Start seated, with knees bent, feet hip-width apart and arms extended out in front of you at shoulder height.
2. As you inhale, start to tuck your pelvis under and roll backwards with a rounded C-shaped spine, until you reach a point where your feet begin to feel light on the floor.

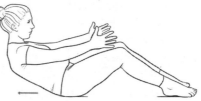

3. Maintain the C-shape you have created and, as you exhale, start to roll back up towards your start position.
4. Repeat.

TIP: Once you have created a C-shaped spine, aim to maintain it as you roll backwards and forwards. This will require your abdominals to work (to prevent you coming out of flexion) and will encourage your hip flexors to move you back and forth (which is what you are after).

REGRESSION: if your arms start to feel too heavy, or the muscles at the base of your neck and across your shoulders (your upper traps) start to feel tight and uncomfortable, you can cross your arms over your chest instead. Reduce the range of movement of the roll back to a point that is manageable for you.

PROGRESSION: you can reach your arms up towards the ceiling to add extra weight to your roll back. You could also try doing this exercise with your legs in tabletop – but do keep them still as you move your pelvis and spine.

Roll ups (suitable for TTC, pregnancy weeks 0–6 and 7–12, and postnatal phase 2)

Roll ups require a good amount of spine mobility, core strength and hip flexor control. They also require concentration and practice! These are all reasons why they are a favourite of mine.

1. Start by lying on your back, with your legs extended and ankles flexed, arms overhead and a neutral spine (don't pop your ribs out).

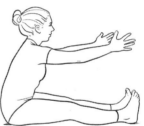

2. As you inhale, start to reach your arms up towards the ceiling, give your head a little nod and begin to peel your spine away from the floor.

3. As you exhale, continue to roll up, aiming to eventually reach forwards to your toes, with your body flexed over your legs.

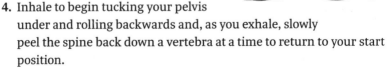

4. Inhale to begin tucking your pelvis under and rolling backwards and, as you exhale, slowly peel the spine back down a vertebra at a time to return to your start position.

TIP: This exercise is all about control and moving through the spine, one vertebra at a time; but in reality, that is really tricky. You'll notice areas of the spine that may move as one big chunk – that's where you should aim to slow things down and take your time.

REGRESSION: try doing the exercise with your knees bent, as this can help to open up the postural chain. You can also try it with a resistance band, holding an end in each hand, and hooking it over the feet. When you get stuck rolling up, you can use your arms to help pull you up, and the band can also help to control you as you roll back down.

PROGRESSION: the slower you move here, the harder the exercise becomes, so go slow. You can also try to keep your arms by your ears throughout.

Side bends (suitable for TTC, entire pregnancy, if comfortable, and postnatal phase 2)

This is a fantastic challenge for shoulder stability, oblique strength and flexibility. It also encourages lateral flexion of the spine, which most of us don't get enough of.

1. Start in a side-sitting position (resting on your right bum cheek, facing the wall rather than the ceiling), with your right hand on the mat underneath your shoulder and in line with your hips. Both knees should be bent, with your left knee pointing upwards and your left foot resting in front of your right (to hold it in place).
2. As you inhale, press into your right hand, push down into your feet, lift your hips up towards the ceiling and aim to straighten the legs and squeeze them together.
3. Exhale to slowly bend the knees and control the release back to the start position. Repeat as required.
4. Follow the same steps, but on your left-hand side.

TIP: You are aiming to come up into a rainbow shape here, not a side plank. This means you need to lift those hips as high as you can manage and shorten the side of the waist. Try not to sink into your shoulder, and I would encourage a soft elbow, so you don't hyperextend your elbow joint.

REGRESSION: you can keep your knees on the floor here, and simply lift the hips up. This means that your rainbow shape will go from knee to hand, rather than feet to hand.

PROGRESSION: this is such a challenging exercise already, so I would focus on nailing the technique, rather than trying to make it harder.

Breaststroke prep (suitable for TTC, pregnancy weeks 0–6 and postnatal phases 1 and 2)

I love breaststroke prep, as it targets the upper back and promotes spine extension. Modern-day lifestyles mean we spend much of our day flexed over laptops, phones, steering wheels, and so we often need to balance this out with exercises like this one.

1. Start by lying on your front, legs a little wider than hip-width apart and in turnout (knees and toes pointing outwards).
2. Place your hands under your forehead, one on top of the other, like a pillow. Aim for a neutral pelvis here (try not to stick your tailbone up in the air too much).
3. Inhale to prepare and, as you exhale, start to gently lift your chest and head, bringing your hands with you, away from the floor so that your body is in a long, low line. Gently press the feet into the floor.
4. Inhale to release back down with control.
5. Repeat.

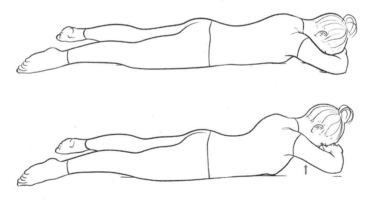

TIP: This is about thoracic-spine extension, which means that the upper back should flatten/straighten slightly – it's not a massive back bend. Think about coming up into a long, low line, rather than trying to get your head up to touch the ceiling.

REGRESSION: keep your hands on the floor and use them to gently help lift you up, rather than pressed against your forehead as you lift.

PROGRESSION: instead of keeping your hands against your forehead like a pillow, try reaching your arms forward in line with the ears and keeping them there as you move. You'll find that the lift feels heavier.

Sweat exercises

Monkey walk (suitable for TTC, entire pregnancy, if comfortable, and postnatal phase 2)

This exercise incorporates a roll down (which I always love) with a plank, and encourages spine mobility, shoulder endurance and core strength.

1. Stand at the end of your mat.
2. Roll down to bring your hands to the floor (you can bend your knees if you need to).
3. Walk out to a plank position.
4. Walk your hands back to your feet, and then roll back up to standing.

TIP: Try not to wiggle your bottom from side to side as you walk out and back in from your plank.

REGRESSION: you can reduce the range of movement, so that you don't walk out to a full-plank each time; or you could remove the roll down/roll up section entirely.

PROGRESSION: add in a push-up when in your full-plank position, before walking back in.

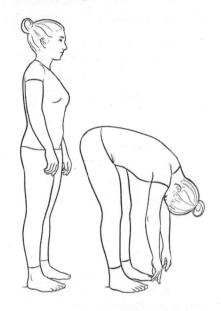

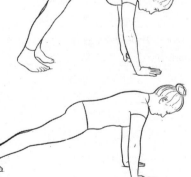

Mountain climbers (suitable for TTC, entire pregnancy, if comfortable, and postnatal phase 2)

Not everyone's favourite
(sorry), but a great endurance
exercise for the shoulders,
core and hip flexors.

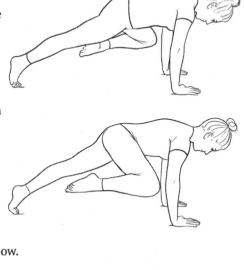

1. Start in a full-plank
   position, with hands
   and feet shoulder-width
   apart, and a nice
   neutral line from head
   to toe.
2. Bring your left knee up
   towards your left elbow.
3. Switch the legs over,
   bringing the right knee
   up towards the right elbow.
4. Repeat.

TIP: The aim is to only ever have one foot on the floor at a time – so it's jumping from one foot to the other in a fast, smooth movement. Try to keep your hips level as you do this, rather than rotating side to side.

REGRESSION: you can do this in a half-plank position, slowing it down and bringing your left knee to your left elbow before replacing it down and then bringing your right knee to your right elbow.

PROGRESSION: pick up the pace and really try to drive the knee as close to the elbow as possible (or towards your chin, if you want to work even harder).

Starbursts (suitable for TTC and pregnancy weeks 0–6 and 7–12)

These are like jumping jacks with a sugar rush. It's a real challenge for leg endurance and will raise the heart rate quickly.

1. Start in a low squat position, with your legs in turnout, heels connected and hands reaching towards the floor.
2. Jump up, reaching the arms and legs out into a star position, before landing as softly as you can and coming back to your start position.
3. Repeat.

TIP: This requires an explosive movement, but do try to land softly (this is much harder).

REGRESSION: remove the jumping element – so essentially, you stand up with your arms extended out to the sides, and then squat back down to your start position.

PROGRESSION: pick up the pace, jump higher or add some dumbbells in your hands for extra resistance.

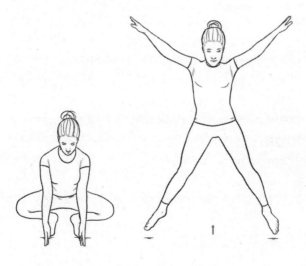

Plankouts (suitable for TTC, pregnancy weeks 0–6, 7–12, 13–19 and 20–27, if comfortable, and postnatal phase 2)

These challenge your plank ability and are pretty advanced. If you're struggling to maintain good technique, please avoid them, as they can aggravate your lower back.

1. Start in a full-plank position, with hands and feet shoulder-width apart, and a nice, neutral line from head to toe.
2. Jump the feet out to slightly wider than your mat, before jumping them back to the start position.
3. Repeat.

TIP: Try to maintain a really strong plank position as the legs move. What you don't want is for the hips to drop lower than the neutral line, as this compresses the lower back.

REGRESSION: rather than jumping both feet out wide each time, try instead to step one foot out at a time, and then one foot back in at a time. This will remove some of the impact and make it easier to maintain a good plank technique.

PROGRESSION: pick up the pace or take the feet wider on the jump out.

Monkey ropes (suitable for TTC, pregnancy weeks 0–6, 7–12, 13–19 and 20–27, if comfortable, and postnatal phase 2)

A real challenge for the core and hip flexors, and an opportunity for some spine flexion.

1. Start seated, with knees bent and feet on the floor.
2. Round your spine slightly, lean back and pick your feet up off the floor, so the legs hover in the air. Reach your arms up and then start to climb, like a monkey on a rope or a fireman on a pole.

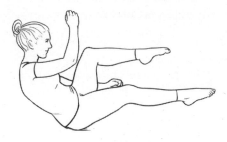

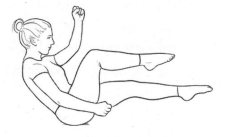

TIP: Try to maintain the slightly rounded spine you have created using your abdominals, while your hip flexors control the movement of the legs. You're aiming to sit on the back of your sit bones here, and the further you lean back, the harder this becomes.

REGRESSION: you can keep your feet on the floor and just climb with the arms.

PROGRESSION: climb faster, lean back further or add weights in the hands for extra resistance.

Example routines

Below, you'll find two example routines. Routine 1 combines all of the exercise options. Routine 2 combines all of the Sweat exercises with a rest period (which you do not have to utilise). Feel free to repeat the routines to help you build up to the recommended 150 minutes of physical activity per week (an example week could be 5 x 30 minute workouts).

Routine 1

- *Warm-up*
- Monkey walk: 30–60 seconds
- Criss-crosses: 30–60 seconds
- Mountain climbers: 30–60 seconds
- Half-roll backs: 30–60 seconds
- Starbursts: 30–60 seconds
- Roll ups: 30–60 seconds
- Plankouts: 30–60 seconds
- Side bends: 30–60 seconds
- Monkey ropes: 30–60 seconds
- Breaststroke prep: 30–60 seconds
- *Repeat or cool-down (if repeating, don't exceed four sets and be sure to include a rest period if you need it between sets)*

Routine 2

- *Warm-up*
- Monkey walk: 30–60 seconds
- Rest – marching on the spot: 60 seconds
- Mountain climbers: 30–60 seconds

- Rest – marching on the spot: 60 seconds
- Starbursts: 30–60 seconds
- Rest – marching on the spot: 60 seconds
- Plankouts: 30–60 seconds
- Rest – marching on the spot: 60 seconds
- Monkey ropes: 30–60 seconds
- *Repeat or cool-down (if repeating, don't exceed four sets and be sure to include a rest period if you need it between sets)*

Your pelvic floor exercise

Blueberries

Bump Plan members often state that this is one of their favourite pelvic floor visualisations, as it really works for them – and to be honest, it's also one of mine. I hope you find it helpful, too, and once you have practised it, you can use it to help you perform other pelvic floor exercises.

1. Start in a comfortable position – this might be seated, lying, side-lying or standing, although seated is usually easiest for this (it'll make sense why in a moment).
2. Close your eyes (this will help you to focus internally) and try to clear your mind.
3. Focus on your breathing by bringing your awareness to breathing in and out through your nose. Relax your jaw and ensure your tongue is relaxed in your mouth.
4. Imagine there is a blueberry on the floor below you (see why a seated position makes sense here?). Inhale and, as you exhale, imagine you are picking the blueberry up off the floor with your vagina. (This will encourage you to both squeeze *and* lift the pelvic floor – which is the absolute goal here.)
5. Inhale to allow the blueberry to drop back to the floor (remember, you're releasing it, not firing it out of a gun!) and then exhale to repeat.
6. Repeat 8–10 times and then rest.

TIP: I like to imagine there is just one blueberry here to pick up to keep it simple, but you could visualise three, and imagine picking one up with each hole (the urethra, vaginal opening and anus) at once.

A guide to nutrition during pregnancy

by Chantal Cuthers, registered nutritionist specialising in fertility, reproductive and infant nutrition

We know that nutrition during pre-conception and pregnancy can provide the foundations for long-term health benefits for your child, support healthy development of the egg and sperm and a healthy embryo and influence a number of health risks across the lifespan. No pressure, right? But having navigated all the information, nervously taken that pregnancy test, checked and rechecked it, you're excitedly pregnant.

It seems that as soon you become pregnant, your body and everything you put in it are in the public domain. Protecting yourself and trying to balance out some decent eating habits, while also ensuring a healthy relationship with food and your body can feel like a giant undertaking. So let's spend a little bit of time on some of the ways you can support your growing body and baby throughout those 40-ish weeks.

The first trimester can really feel all about survival. For those who are not blessed with that glow, and instead just feel constipated, while the food aversions come in thick and fast, it's important to understand that sometimes it's simply about ensuring adequate food and fluid intake, and not focusing on the details. Nausea tips includes keeping your stomach from getting empty – crackers by the bed when you wake, small and frequent snacks, and vitamin B6 can be helpful.

The second trimester can offer a reprieve for many, so this is where you can focus on some solid nutrition for the rest of your pregnancy. Try to ensure you have regular and consistent meals and snacks with a focus on varied ingredients to ensure a variety of nutrients that come from different foods. If you're not allergic yourself, it can be helpful to expose your baby to common allergen foods such as cooked fish, nuts, dairy, eggs and soy by eating them now.

The third trimester can be a combination of finally getting the hang of the food and not having enough stomach space to eat it. Keep meals small and frequent, sit upright for some time after eating and focus on plenty of variety where you can.

Food behaviours for pregnancy

Pregnancy is a time when so little feels in your control, so being able to make some food choices that serve you outside of just nutrition is key.

Here are some questions to consider when pregnant and supporting your body:

- Are you eating regular meals and snacks or does coffee creep in as breakfast frequently?
- Are you eating enough day to day, and are you removing distractions, such as the office computer, phone and TV while you eat, where possible?
- Are you including foods you enjoy with a range of foods that are helpful to your body in this moment?
- Are you finding time to switch off, connect with yourself, your friends, your partner?
- What does your movement look like – restorative, stress reducing, meditative; or high intensity, without recovery and low on fuel afterwards?

What about weight?

Weight stigma and fatphobia cause a lot of damage in the fertility and pregnancy space, with even some health professionals ignoring the indisputable evidence around the damage of intentional weight loss, at a time when the focus should be on nourishment and not restriction.

When it comes to having a well-nourished body for pre-conception needs and the sheer energy required to grow a baby, we need to insure would-be parents don't restrict and instead take any opportunity to add or aid nutrition. Of course, if there are foods you're intolerant to or are a risk to your baby and pregnancy you want to avoid these, but all safe foods should be accessed to support your overwhelming energy needs now and in preparation for labour and birth. Your body will gain the weight it needs to gain, driven by genetics and the individual pregnancy itself and you will have very little control over this.

Nutrition concerns in pregnancy that likely require specialised support are gestational diabetes, preeclampsia, iron deficiency or anaemia.

Let's take a look at the key nutrients to support a healthy pregnancy.

Folate

This is the only nutrient recommended worldwide for pre-conception and pregnancy (the recommended dose varies slightly depending on country). It is crucial for the growth and development of your baby, including DNA, cells, spinal cord and brain. You can get it from cooked eggs, dark green leafy vegetables (like spinach, kale and broccoli), berries, avocados, seeds and nuts, but because food sources are not so bioavailable (easy to absorb and utilise), please ensure you're taking a minimum of 400mcg of folic acid supplements, and topping it up with an activated folate like methyl folate in line with your health provider's advice, especially if you have a history of miscarriage, MTHFR gene mutations, a family history of neural tube defects (NTDs), IBD, coeliac, diabetes, a previous pregnancy affected by an NTD or you're on long-term medications (including epilepsy meds and HIV antivirals). Take folic acid at least 1 month prior to conception and through the first trimester, and if you do tick any of the at-risk markers, the advice is usually to take up to 5000mcg daily (seek the advice and support of your health provider with this).

Iodine

Usually required to supplement throughout pregnancy and breastfeeding; however, if you have a thyroid condition, please consult with your healthcare team. Iodine is crucial for the baby's brain and nervous system development, and for maintaining thyroid function in the birthing parent to ensure that body temperature and metabolic needs are regulated. Dietary sources include iodised salt, kelp, seaweed, cooked fish and seafood. The guideline for supplementation is 150mg daily – but be aware that if you're on a prenatal supplement containing iodine, you should not take additional iodine supplements.

Iron

Iron needs in pregnancy increase, as 30 per cent of your total blood volume is needed to create blood for baby. We know low healthy iron status increases risk of fatigue, maternal iron deficiency or anaemia and low birthweight babies. Iron levels are also notoriously low in menstruating folk, so most are already deficient before heading into pregnancy.

Cooked red meat, eggs, legumes that have been well prepared and green leafy veg are all great options. It's about small but more regular portions for absorption, rather than eating one iron-rich meal per day. Adding vitamin-C-rich foods like red bell pepper and citrus will also help absorption. If you're low or in the lower range of normal in ferritin tests, it might be worth chatting to your healthcare provider about iron supplementation. Some options can cause constipation, while others that are more gentle may take longer to replenish your levels and cost a little more, but should still be considered. It's recommended that most people take an iron supplement every second day.

Choline

The more we research this, the more we understand it to be just as crucial as folate for spinal cord building and brain function. It is found in egg yolks especially, soy, peanuts and some meat and fish. Make sure your prenatal supplement contains choline if you're taking one, especially if you do not consume eggs as a daily part of your diet (if you do, two cooked eggs per day is a great foundation). However, most prenatal and pregnancy supplements do not contain choline so you might need to supplement with 440mcg daily, but consult your health provider first.

Calcium

Required for growing a healthy baby and bone structure – but did you know it's far more crucial in the second half of pregnancy to ensure you're getting extra, so that your own bones aren't broken down to fuel baby's growth. Great sources are fish bones from small fish, green leafy veg, almonds, tofu, sesame seeds, full-fat dairy. Supplementation is not usually required, but vitamin D3/K2 supplementation can help to support your absorption and utilisation if you're deemed high risk or can't consume dairy products.

Vitamin D

This hormone-like vitamin is crucial for baby's growth, nerve and muscle cells and to reduce the risk of pregnancy complications. If you can eat extra mushrooms, oily fish and egg yolk, combined with getting plenty of morning sunshine on as much skin as possible through summer (without burning), then this is a good start. Vitamin D supplementation should be a part of any UK winter prescription at 10mcg daily from September through March, and throughout the whole year for those with darker skin, anyone who wears cultural or religious coverings such as hijab or veils, those who avoid the sunshine strictly for medical reasons or who have medications that affect vitamin D levels. It works with phosphate and calcium when pregnant for development of bones, teeth and lowering the risk of eczema and preterm birth. Supplementation can be funded through the NHS in the UK.

Vitamin B12

You cannot get this from plant foods, so you need to eat animal products, nutritional yeast, products such as cereals and plant milks that have been fortified with B12 or take a supplement. My top food sources are organic or grass-fed meats, eggs, cooked fish, and full-fat dairy. This crucial vitamin helps to produce blood cells and DNA and supports early embryo development. A blood test will show whether or not you're getting enough, and supplementing prior to conception might be necessary if your levels are too low.

Zinc

Zinc is important for building immunity and cells in your baby and to ensure you've got some immunity cells functioning too, plus it helps gut strength and mood. Good food sources include eggs, nuts and seeds (especially walnuts and pumpkin seeds) and cooked seafood. Supplement only with the advice of a health professional.

Omega-3 fatty acids (known as DHA and EPA)

Important for healthy brain development and cell structure during gestation, these act as anti-inflammatories and are supportive of healthy egg and sperm function. Linked to a reduction in pre-term birth and increased cognitive development in children, they are found in fatty fish such as sardines and salmon and in much smaller amounts in flaxseed and its oil, walnuts, chia and hemp.

I recommend supplementing with quality DHA/EPA if you don't meet a recommended two to three servings of fatty fish in your meals per week (and unfortunately, plant sources will not meet your pregnancy requirements). You want to look for independently tested omega-3 supplements with a higher DHA:EPA ratio and DHA at 1000mg until 36 weeks, when we stop temporarily to ensure they don't impact when we go into labour. Keep all omega-3 supplements refrigerated after opening.

Note: if you do consume fish, be mindful of avoiding high-mercury varieties, such as tuna, swordfish, marlin, shark – and always avoid raw fish and shellfish.

I'm plant-based – should I focus on anything specific?

Plant-based diets risk being low in iron, B12, vitamin D, choline, omega-3 mostly, and sometimes calcium and zinc, so consult your health provider to ensure you're getting the minimum of what you need.

Food safety in pregnancy

Food safety guidelines are there to protect from any risk of food-borne illnesses that could be dangerous for your pregnancy or baby. While in some cases the risk might be low, the consequences can be high. The NHS has easily accessible information on foods to avoid[16] and these guidelines should be incorporated into your food planning the second you become pregnant (they're updated when needed and may be different from one pregnancy to the next, so always re-check).

When do you need to worry about food intake or sickness in pregnancy?

If you're losing body weight and cannot keep anything down (fluids in particular), you need to check in with your care providers. Sometimes you might need someone to advocate for you and to be very strong with getting you the support you need. Being unable to take care of other children, drive, get to work, losing weight (especially 10 per cent of your pre-pregnancy body weight), being unable to keep fluids down, and having dizzy or lightheaded spells risking balance are not normal. You may need medical attention, fluids and medication to ensure you're safe – so that your baby is safe.

So where to from here?

I want to reiterate the importance of finding a safe and balanced attitude to nourishing your body while not over-thinking every small portion or meal. The reality is that pregnancy can be hard – emotionally, physically and mentally – and there is so much to learn about food safety guidelines and navigating new aversions or cravings. Ensuring you focus on trying to nourish your body and baby in these moments is crucial.

This time can be exciting, overwhelming, challenging, lonely, enjoyable – any or all of these things in one day. What we used to do with the support of a village is now largely left up to couples or singles to attempt alone, so building a great support network around yourself and, while clichéd, looking to things you can control and letting go of what you can't, is very helpful. Finding your feet in pregnancy doesn't always come easily, so being honest with your needs and boundaries is a crucial part of pregnancy wellbeing.

Trust your gut, seek help when you think you need it and try to make space for enjoyable meals, social interaction and a little awareness around the nutrients that will support this journey.

Pregnancy weeks 7–12

I'm presuming that by this stage, you may have taken a few pregnancy tests and seen those two lines, but have yet to have an official dating scan (which in the UK happens around weeks 10–14). This can be a strange time for some, and a lot of hopes can be placed on that first scan, while at the same time not wanting to get *too* excited just yet. I hope that you're managing to feel positive and to enjoy this period, despite any uncertainty (and particularly if you've experienced a previous loss).

As I was actively trying to conceive, I knew I was pregnant by now and continued to train in the same way that I had preconception, following the UK CMOs' guidelines on physical activity during pregnancy. This meant that it was an easy transition for me; but if you haven't viewed those guidelines yet, please do head now to p. 24. What I found most difficult was the sheer exhaustion and lack of energy that hit me as soon as I fell pregnant. I'm always so shocked at how quickly these symptoms kick in, so I hope you're coping!

Your body

While this stage of pregnancy can still feel very 'early days', for many, the symptoms will have definitely arrived. These can feel both reassuring and tough at the same time, so do be kind to yourself. I know that many people don't feel comfortable sharing their pregnancy news until after their first scan, but I personally feel it's worth confiding in those close to you, so they can help you through what can sometimes be the hardest period of pregnancy.

Here are some of the most common symptoms during this phase:

- **Extreme tiredness/exhaustion.** This is particularly prevalent in the first trimester, which seems all the more cruel, as you may not have told colleagues or friends at this point. I would nod off at the drop of a hat, but luckily, I only share my office with my husband. You may find your motivation to exercise slips here, but don't panic – for most people it will come back.
- **Nausea and/or pregnancy sickness.** This can fall anywhere on a spectrum from very mild to an incredibly debilitating version called hyperemesis gravidarum. For more on this, and where to get support, see p. 142.
- **Sore boobs.** Another one to thank your hormones for, this is often one of the earliest symptoms that alerts you to pregnancy. Make sure you invest now in a good sports bra – there are so many available that cater to pregnancy and the postpartum period.

- **The need to urinate more often.** At this stage, this is in response to pregnancy hormones (later in pregnancy, it'll also be due to pressure on your bladder as your uterus grows).
- **An alteration/intensifying of emotions.** If anyone told me the way I was feeling was because of my hormones I wanted to bite their head off, but sadly, it turns out our hormones do affect our moods from early on.

While our little ones may be tiny, by week 12, a foetus is fully formed, with all organs, muscles, bones and limbs in place, and now their main job is to get bigger. That's pretty impressive, right?

What you need to know

The reasons I most often hear for why someone may not be particularly active at this stage are the sheer exhaustion or nausea that can come as quite a shock. I remember having such low energy and motivation at times, and I suffered with nausea and vomiting in the first 16 weeks.

For many women, if they can encourage themselves into sports clothes, and peel themselves away from the sofa, exercise can make symptoms feel more manageable. Of course, no two pregnancies feel the same, so I don't want to overpromise, but it really is worth keeping this in mind. Physical activity can boost mood, improve sleep (not the duration, necessarily, but the quality) and may just help to shake some of the lethargy you feel. Overall, I would say don't berate yourself if you find your motivation to move is lacking – for many it will resume. The first trimester is tough – hang in there!

What can I do on those low-energy days?

On days when you want to do something that will strengthen or benefit your body, but you have zero energy, you might want to consider some breathwork. I know, I know, you're probably thinking that you breathe without even thinking about it, so why would you bother with breathwork? And yes, it can sound a bit hippy-dippy, but practising breathwork is essentially giving your diaphragm (your main breathing muscle) a workout; it does for your diaphragm what squats do for your glutes – and as your main breathing muscle, the diaphragm is seriously important (and, sadly, often forgotten about).

To understand why breathwork is so important, let's first discuss the mechanisms of regular breathing.

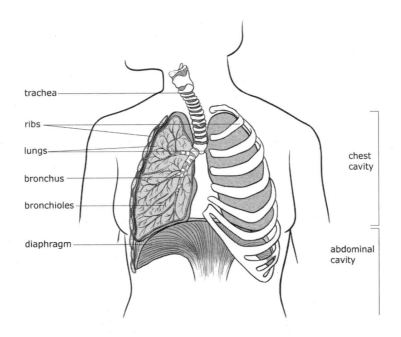

The diaphragm is shaped like an upside-down bowl or beanie hat, nestled within the ribcage. It separates the chest cavity from the abdominal cavity and is responsible for your inhale. When the diaphragm contracts, it flattens downwards becoming more of a plate shape, and creates a vacuum in the lungs. This sucks air into the lungs; hence you inhale. When the diaphragm then relaxes, it moves back into its curved shape, and air is forced back out of the lungs, hence you exhale.

This all happens automatically – you don't sit on the sofa watching TV while thinking 'inhale, exhale, inhale, exhale'. However, ideally, you want the diaphragm to be the primary muscle doing the work, and you may find sometimes that secondary muscles in the chest and neck can take over and try to help, or even do most of the work. These muscles are not as efficient, and using them can cause tension in the neck, so you want the diaphragm to do the work.

Breathwork is essentially focused-breathing practice. It encourages you to use the diaphragm to breathe and, in so doing, it should get stronger and perform its job better – a win–win!

An extra bonus is that studies suggest that diaphragmatic breathing can help to lower cortisol levels (a stress hormone), reduce anxiety and depression, lower blood pressure and stimulate the vagus nerve, which helps to dial up the 'rest-and-digest' system.[17, 18, 19] The 'rest-and-digest' system is another name for the parasympathetic nervous system and can be thought of as the opposite of the 'fight-or-flight' system. It's responsible for many of the body's automatic functions and can reduce heart rate, increase rate of digestion, slow breathing and more, to help you relax and recuperate after a stressful or dangerous situation.

How to practice diaphragmatic breathing

1. Make sure you are sitting, lying or standing comfortably. Personally, I like doing this in a seated or side-lying position.
2. Begin by inhaling through your nose and exhaling through your mouth. Get this circular pattern of breathing started first.
3. With each inhale, start to visualise the diaphragm contracting, and sucking air into the lungs, until there is no space left.
4. On the exhale, imagine the diaphragm relaxing, and all the air from the lungs being emptied out; keep exhaling, until there is no more air left in the lungs.
5. Start to notice how the core expands on the inhale (this is due to pressure changes in the area, which we'll discuss later) and relaxes as you exhale.
6. As you inhale, imagine the ribcage expanding in all directions (out to the sides, front and back), and on the exhale, notice it contracting back inwards.
7. Continue for up to 5 minutes and then relax and breathe in your normal fashion.

This is a practice you could perform daily and becomes even more important as you progress through pregnancy. As your uterus grows upwards, it gets closer to the diaphragm and can make it more difficult to breathe deeply, so regular practice can help you to stay on top of your breathing technique and diaphragm strength.

What is the focus in weeks 7-12?

As is the case throughout your pregnancy, you will be aiming to meet the UK CMOs' guidelines for physical activity during pregnancy (see p. 24). These will stay the same until you give birth, but will look different as your symptoms vary, energy levels adapt and bump size alters over the coming months. Essentially, you want to continue combining at least 150 minutes of cardiovascular exercise with musculoskeletal exercise, at a level where you can still talk.

As with the start of the first trimester, you can still make the most of not having a large bump yet and get in some functional core work that should help to give you a more comfortable and more supportive pregnancy. Ensuring that the muscles of the core are 'showing up to the party' now is a really good idea. That's why there are some important exercises for your core in the Strength workout in this phase.

I'd also start prioritising your pelvic floor workouts (see this chapter's pelvic floor exercise on p. 140). As the uterus gets bigger, it gets heavier, and the demand it places on the pelvic floor increases. This is because one of its main roles is to support the weight of the pelvic organs – the uterus being one of these. Again, starting pregnancy with a strong, functional pelvic floor can reduce the chances of pelvic floor dysfunction (such as stress incontinence or pelvic organ prolapse) further down the line.

Your exercises: weeks 7–12

Your warm-up and cool-down exercises can be found on pp. 74–76 and 87–88. Now let's go through the exercises for the second half of your first trimester.

Strength exercises

Single leg stretches (suitable for TTC, pregnancy weeks 0–6 and 7–12 and postnatal phase 2)

Single leg stretches are great for improving abdominal endurance and hip flexor strength.

1. Start lying on your back, legs in a tabletop position, fingers to temples and elbows wide.
2. Lift your head and shoulders gently away from the mat, so your upper back is flexed.
3. Inhale and then, as you exhale, extend your left leg out as low as you can, keeping your pelvis neutral.
4. Inhale to switch the legs over and exhale to extend the right leg out as low as you can, keeping the pelvis neutral.
5. Repeat.

TIP: Aim to maintain a neutral pelvis throughout, only allowing the legs to dip as low as you can manage. The legs move constantly, almost like you are riding a bike (rather than coming back to tabletop between each leg extension).

REGRESSION: you can do this with your head and shoulders in contact with the mat, rather than lifted. Aim to keep a neutral spine, though – don't allow your lower back to aggressively arch away from the floor.

PROGRESSION: reach your arms up towards the ceiling/alongside your ears; this will add weight to your abdominals.

Hip circles (suitable for TTC, entire pregnancy, if comfortable, and postnatal phase 2)

This exercise is quite challenging, requiring a good amount of core stability and hip flexor control. Only continue during pregnancy if you are managing the core pressure well (see p. 174).

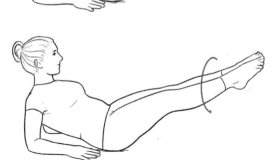

1. Start seated, resting back on your forearms, with your legs in a tabletop position and your spine in neutral.
2. Extend your legs up, imagining that your feet are pointing to the number twelve on a clock.
3. Inhale to begin circling the legs around your imaginary clock (clockwise) towards the number six, then exhale to continue the circle back to twelve.
4. Repeat anticlockwise.

TIP: The aim here is to keep the pelvis as still as possible, while the legs draw their circles. The spine should not be flexing and extending; it should stay stable.

REGRESSION: try doing this with slightly bent knees, or with the legs in tabletop. You are still aiming to move the legs in a circle, but they will not feel as heavy.

PROGRESSION: simply draw bigger circles, taking them as big as you can, keeping your pelvis still.

Dead bugs (suitable for TTC, pregnancy weeks 0–6 and 7–12 and postnatal phase 2)

Dead bugs are another one of my favourite stability exercises. They look so simple, but to maintain a neutral spine as the limbs move requires control and concentration.

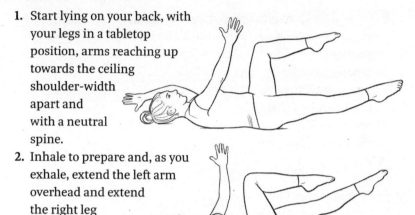

1. Start lying on your back, with your legs in a tabletop position, arms reaching up towards the ceiling shoulder-width apart and with a neutral spine.

2. Inhale to prepare and, as you exhale, extend the left arm overhead and extend the right leg towards the end of your mat, as low as you can maintain a neutral spine (don't let the ribcage pop up, or the lower back aggressively arch away from the floor).

3. Inhale to return to the start, and then exhale as you extend the right arm and left leg.

4. Inhale to return.

5. Repeat.

TIP: The aim here is to keep the spine and pelvis stable and still as the limbs move. Think about hugging your ribcage into the body to prevent your spine extending as you open out, and only allow the leg and arm to drop as low as you can maintain your position.

REGRESSION: rather than moving both an arm and a leg at the same time, just choose one. So maybe you only move the arms at first, until you feel stronger, and then you only move the legs. Slowly build up to moving both.

PROGRESSION: take both legs, or both arms or all four limbs away from each other as you exhale. This requires a lot of control, so start with a smaller range of movement and gradually build up.

Half- to full-planks (suitable for TTC, entire pregnancy, if comfortable, and postnatal phase 2)

This is a great exercise for encouraging good full-plank technique and, if continued in pregnancy, you can stop when the full-plank becomes too much and simply practise your half-plank endurance instead.

1. Start in a half-plank position, with knees hip-width apart, hands shoulder-width apart, and a nice, neutral line from your ears to your knees.
2. Inhale to prepare and, as you exhale, float the knees up off the floor, until you are in a full-plank position.
3. Inhale to float the knees back to the floor to half-plank.
4. Repeat.

TIP: Try not to sink into your arms, as they will take a fair amount of the weight here. Think about pressing into your little fingers to help activate the serratus anterior muscles at the sides of your ribs. We want a nice, neutral line here whether in the half- or full-plank position.

REGRESSION: simply practise – and nail – your half-plank position.

PROGRESSION: start in full-plank position. Exhale to lift your hips up into the air, folding at the hips, creating a triangle shape with your body. Inhale to lower the hips slowly back down to a full-plank position.

Glute bridges (suitable for TTC, pregnancy weeks 0–6 and 7–12 and postnatal phases 1 and 2)

Performed correctly, glute bridges are a great way to activate the glute muscles and lengthen the hip flexors. When you spend a lot of time seated, they are perfect for balancing you out.

1. Start lying on your back with a neutral spine and pelvis, knees bent, feet hip-width apart and arms extended up towards the ceiling.
2. Inhale to prepare, and as you exhale, press down into the feet and start to lift the hips up into the air, until you have a nice, neutral line from the ribcage to the knees.
3. Inhale to stay, and then exhale to lower back to the start position with control.
4. Repeat.

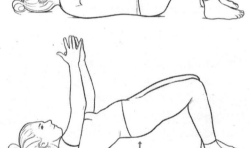

TIP: You are aiming to keep the neutral line you have created as you lift and lower the hips. If you tuck your pelvis under (a posterior tilt) as you lift your hips up, you may experience cramp in your hamstrings. If you do the opposite and stick your bottom out (an anterior tilt) as you lift up your hips, your lower back may feel tight. Instead, you want the pelvis to stay neutral, and for the glutes to do the work.

REGRESSION: have your arms by your side, palms down, so you can use them for stability as you lift the hips. You could also reduce the range of movement, and only take the hips a few inches away from the floor.

PROGRESSION: take your arms overhead, without allowing your ribcage to flare, which requires more abdominal control. You can also tie a resistance band or loop around your knees to press out on to; or put a yoga block or ball between your knees to squeeze into.

Sweat exercises

High knees (suitable for TTC, entire pregnancy, if comfortable, and postnatal phase 2)

This is essentially jogging on the spot, but with more demand on the hip flexors and cardiovascular system.

1. Starting from a standing position, begin jogging on the spot.
2. Put your hands out in front of you at hip height, palms down, and gradually take the knees higher and higher, until they hit your hands.

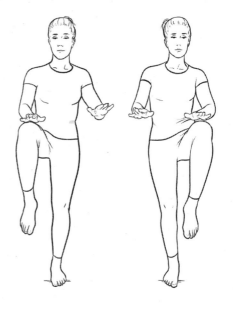

TIP: You may be tempted to lean back a little here but avoid doing so too much, as this can make your lower back unhappy. Try to be as bouncy and springy as possible as you do this to really activate the calf muscles.

REGRESSION: instead of starting with jogging, start by marching on the spot. This way, you still have the same height to bring the leg up to, but less impact and bounce are needed.

PROGRESSION: pick up the pace; or try to take the knees even higher.

Planks to squats (suitable for TTC and pregnancy weeks 0–6 and 7–12)

This is a bit of a spicy one that challenges shoulder, core and leg strength . . . you've been warned!

1. Start in a full-plank position, hands shoulder-width apart, and a nice, neutral line from ear to ankle.
2. Jump your feet up towards your hands, landing in a squat position with your bottom low and then bring your arms up, so they are extended out in front of you.
3. Put your hands back on the floor and jump back into your full-plank position.
4. Repeat.

TIP: This should be an explosive but smooth movement. You'll need a fair amount of hip mobility to get your feet into your squat position. Make sure your full-plank position is strong when you jump out – don't let the hips drop too low.

REGRESSION: you can step your feet forwards, one at a time, to bring yourself into your squat position, and then step out one foot at a time into your plank position (rather than jumping).

PROGRESSION: try to take your hands off the floor before your feet touch it (so there's almost a moment when you are totally off the floor). This requires speed and agility – and is very tricky!

Hand slaps (suitable for TTC, entire pregnancy, if comfortable, and postnatal phase 2)

This challenges your ability to keep your pelvis stable as you lose your base of support (one of your arms). A great exercise to target the transversus abdominis and pelvic floor (your main pelvis and lower back stabilisers).

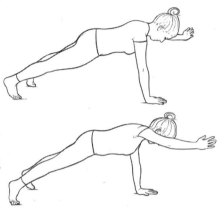

1. Start in a half- or full-plank position, hands shoulder-width apart and knees or feet hip-width apart.
2. Imagine that there is a fly in front of your face, hassling you, and with your left hand try to slap it away.
3. Switch and use your right hand to try to slap it away.

TIP: The aim of this exercise is to try to keep the spine and pelvis still while the arms are moving. The normal reaction is for the pelvis to rotate slightly, or to sink into the supporting arm, so try to avoid this by switching on your stabilisers.

REGRESSION: take the knees or feet wider to give you a better base of support and make it easier to keep the pelvis stable. You could also try simply lifting the hand a few centimetres off the floor, rather than swatting away the fly, before replacing it and switching to the other hand.

PROGRESSION: reach further forwards with the arm, as if the fly is far away from you.

Tombstones (suitable for TTC and pregnancy weeks 0–6 and 7–12)

I love this exercise, as it feels really bouncy, explosive and dynamic. It's not an easy one, but it's definitely fun!

1. Start lying on your back with your arms extended overhead (by your ears), legs extended along the mat and a neutral spine.
2. Reach your arms up towards the ceiling and curl up to seated (almost like you're doing a roll up).
3. Using your hands to help (if needed), stand up and jump up into the air with arms reaching overhead.
4. Squat down, until your bum is on the floor (again, use your hands, if needed) and lie back down on your back, returning to your start position.
5. Repeat.

TIP: Do not be afraid to use your hands here for support when coming up to standing (it's tricky without them); and some people find it easier if they cross their legs over on the way up, too.

REGRESSION: slow it down. While this exercise is designed to be fast and explosive, do reduce the pace, and feel free to remove the jump, too, while you are getting the hang of it.

PROGRESSION: pick up the pace. It's already a tricky exercise, so speed is your friend here; and you could try *not* using your hands to help, if you are feeling really brave.

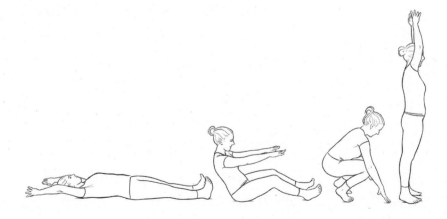

Sprints (suitable for TTC, pregnancy weeks 0–6 and 7–12 and postnatal phase 2)

This really does what it says on the tin and needs little description here – but it is a great way to increase your heart rate.

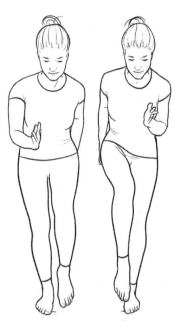

1. Start in a standing position and begin jogging on the spot.
2. Start to increase the pace, until you are sprinting on the spot, with your arms moving, too.

TIP: Think about landing quietly – I like to imagine there's a sleeping dog in the room that I don't want to wake. It's harder and builds calf strength, too.

REGRESSION: simply slow it down to a jog.

PROGRESSION: simply pick up the pace; or you could add some dumbbells into the hands for extra resistance.

Example routines

Below, you'll find two example routines. Routine 1 combines all of the exercise options. Routine 2 combines all of the Sweat exercises with a rest period (which you do not have to utilise). Feel free to repeat the routines to help you build up to the recommended 150 minutes of physical activity per week (an example week could be 5 x 30 minute workouts).

Routine 1

- *Warm-up*
- High knees: 30–60 seconds
- Single leg stretches: 30–60 seconds
- Planks to squats: 30–60 seconds
- Hip circles: 30-60 seconds
- Hand slaps: 30–60 seconds
- Dead bugs: 30–60 seconds
- Tombstones: 30–60 seconds
- Half- to full-planks: 30–60 seconds
- Sprints: 30–60 seconds
- Glute bridges: 30–60 seconds
- *Repeat or cool-down* (if repeating, don't exceed four sets and be sure to include a rest period if you need it between sets)

Routine 2

- *Warm-up*
- High knees: 30–60 seconds
- Rest – marching on the spot: 60 seconds
- Planks to squats: 30–60 seconds

- Rest – marching on the spot: 60 seconds
- Hand slaps: 30–60 seconds
- Rest – marching on the spot: 60 seconds
- Tombstones: 30–60 seconds
- Rest – marching on the spot: 60 seconds
- Sprints: 30–60 seconds
- *Repeat or cool-down* (if repeating, don't exceed four sets and be sure to include a rest period if you need it between sets)

Your pelvic floor exercise

Four corners

If you look back at where the pelvic floor muscles are situated (see p. 52), you can see that they span from the pubic bone at the front of the pelvis to the coccyx at the back and out to the sit bones at the side. I therefore like to imagine that the pelvic floor is a diamond shape with four corners. But for this exercise, I'd like you to go a step further and imagine it as a tissue – again, with four corners, as above.

1. Start in a comfortable position – this might be seated, lying, side-lying, standing.
2. Close your eyes (this will help you to focus internally) and try to clear your mind.
3. Focus on your breathing by bringing your awareness to breathing in and out through your nose. Relax your jaw and ensure your tongue is relaxed in your mouth.
4. Visualise the pelvic floor as a tissue, spanning the base of the pelvis.
5. Start by focusing on the front corner of the tissue. Inhale and then, as you exhale, think about lifting up that front corner using your pelvic floor, and folding it in towards the middle of the tissue.
6. Inhale to release and then exhale to repeat.
7. Repeat 5 times.
8. Repeat the above for each corner in turn (repeating 5 times each).

9. Now, imagine on your exhale, picking the tissue up from the centre, lifting all four corners with it.

10. Release and relax on the inhale, imagining the tissue floating back to its start position.

11. Repeat 5 times.

TIP: Don't worry if the concept or *feeling* of lifting and folding this imaginary tissue seems too much to consider. For most of us, simply lifting the pelvic floor is hard enough. It's really just a goal – something to visualise and aim for. What's most important is that you are moving away from the 'hold-in-a-wee' technique that so many of us have adopted that simply isn't thorough enough. Instead, you want the entire pelvic floor to be activated – front, back and sides.

Nausea, vomiting and hyperemesis gravidarum: navigating tough symptoms

by Dr Caitlin Dean, Chair of the Pregnancy Sickness Support charity

It is well known that feeling and being sick are part and parcel of early pregnancy. For a lot of people, particularly first time around, it is a welcome sign of the pregnancy developing and many women see it as a bit of a rite of passage. For the vast majority, waves of nausea and some occasional vomiting are normal and nothing to worry about. As a result of nausea (and other factors like cutting out alcohol and consciously trying to be healthier), it is common to lose a little bit of weight in the first trimester.

If you are feeling nauseous, try to prevent your stomach from getting empty. Nibbling bland foods like toast or biscuits can help, while resting when it's worse can help to manage it. Also, masking unpleasant smells that trigger your nausea – with essential oils or mint – for example, may help. There are lots of 'remedies' for pregnancy sickness, ranging from sour sweets to acupressure bands you wear on your wrists, but unfortunately, there is no real evidence that any of them work. That said, they are unlikely to cause any harm, so they may be worth trying.

Mention to anyone that you are feeling sick, and you'll be advised to try ginger. Wouldn't it be wonderful if such a simple remedy could stop pregnancy sickness in its tracks and cure us all? Sadly, the evidence for it having any real effect just isn't there; in fact, it can even make symptoms a bit worse, as it can cause heartburn and a burning sensation if it's vomited back up. If you are a fan of ginger generally and it doesn't cause you acid reflux, then by all means, try it – but if you don't much like it in the first place, don't force yourself to take it in the belief that it will make you feel better. A slice of toast is likely to have a greater effect!

For some unlucky people, pregnancy sickness can be much more severe. Some women find the nausea can be unbearably overwhelming and make it difficult to eat or drink or even move. Even if there isn't much (or any) actual vomiting, the nausea can be utterly miserable and have a terrible effect on your life. If you are also vomiting a lot, or if the nausea is so bad that you're not able to eat and drink at all, it can lead to a lot of other problems, such as dehydration and malnutrition. These more extreme types of pregnancy sickness are known as moderate–severe nausea and vomiting of pregnancy and hyperemesis gravidarum (HG).

Symptoms severe enough to affect your day-to-day life, your ability to work or care for your family and are stopping you from eating and drinking as you normally would should be taken seriously. That is not normal pregnancy sickness. Your first port of call for symptoms like this can be your GP or midwife. There is a range of medications which can help and which have been used in pregnancy for decades without any evidence that they cause any harm at all to the baby. In the UK, there is one specifically licensed for nausea and vomiting in pregnancy.

Unfortunately, it is not always that easy to get treatment and those treatments that are available aren't always particularly effective. Some people will get a lot of relief from a single medication, but those suffering with HG often require multiple medications and frequent trips to the hospital for rehydration through a drip. Accessing medication in the first place can also be challenging, as there are a lot of misconceptions and fears about taking medicine in pregnancy.

Decisions about how to treat HG should be based on the balance between the risks and benefits of both taking and not taking treatment. Generally, when it comes to HG, the risks of not taking medication – and therefore not being able to eat and drink, take your pregnancy vitamin and folic acid and the misery and depression it can cause – are far more severe than any hypothetical risk of the medications, which, as previously said, have been used for decades without evidence that they cause specific problems.

For people who don't get relief from medications and require a lot of time in hospital, HG can be a real slog and a very miserable experience. It is normal to have thoughts about terminating your wanted baby when you are suffering so much, and this, in turn, can lead to feelings of guilt and inadequacy as a mother-to-be. People can be very hard on themselves about experiencing these feelings, but it really is not surprising when you are so very unwell.

Reaching out for help and support is key to survival. The UK charity Pregnancy Sickness Support offers a helpline and ongoing peer support, plus a pregnancy-sickness-specific counselling service. We may not have an effective cure for everyone with this condition yet, but we can certainly reduce the misery through proper information and support. If you are more distressed than you expected to be and it is affecting your wellbeing, please reach out for help.

If you have suffered with severe pregnancy sickness, be kind to yourself with regard to recovering. You may find you need to readjust your diet and exercise levels slowly over time if you have been eating and moving very little for months. Take it easy and appreciate that you are recovering from a severe illness.

Pregnancy weeks 13–19

You've hit the second trimester. Fantastic! Now you start to feel fine again, yes? Well, maybe, maybe not.

I remember thinking that at week 12 I would feel like I'd been reborn – I'd no longer feel nauseous, I'd start to glow and I'd have copious amounts of energy. The reality was, however, that I was still ready to eyeball anyone who ate anything 'fragrant' on the underground, and I was still using socks* to wipe my mouth on car journey sick stops (*top tip – always carry tissues).

All jokes aside, 12 weeks is an important milestone for many, especially those who have experienced a previous loss. Your foetus is now fully formed (their organs, muscles, limbs and bones are in place) and, moving forwards, its job is to simply grow and mature. Your risk of miscarriage reduces after this point (80 per cent occur within the first 12 weeks[20]), and hopefully, with that come some feelings of reassurance.

Your body

Between weeks 11 and 13 (in the UK), you'll usually be offered an ultrasound scan, which will mark your first glimpse of your baby, and many people use this as an opportunity to share their big news with the world. While there's so much to be excited about at 12 weeks, it's important to manage your expectations of your symptoms – sadly, it is not a magic number that means all your symptoms disappear. However – and I know you might not thank me for saying it – those symptoms you do experience are a sign of a healthy pregnancy and will hopefully pass soon. Hang in there; you're doing great!

Common symptoms during this phase include:

- **Increased sex drive.** This can be due to pregnancy hormones and/or increased blood flow to the pelvic area. Please note that some of us (including me) will have a decrease in sex drive, and that is understandable, too.
- **Increased discharge.** This should be thin and clear or milky in appearance. If it has a pungent smell or you are itchy or sore, do let your midwife know.
- **Constipation.** There are various reasons why you may experience constipation during pregnancy. The body slows down the passage of food through the intestines to access as many nutrients as possible from it, plus it removes more water, thus drying it out. Further along in pregnancy, you may find that your enlarged uterus also plays a role. Try increasing your fibre and water intake, be more active (often the answer) and speak to your GP if you are struggling. It might also be worth investing in a 'squatty potty' or small stool (excuse the pun) to elevate your feet when pooing, as this can help you to empty your bowels fully.
- **Round ligament pain.** This is usually experienced as short, sharp spasms in your lower bump or groin area that can come as a bit of a shock. While harmless, it is caused by

stretching of the uterus and surrounding ligaments and is often described as feeling almost like an elastic band snapping. If you experience this during a workout, I'd advise you to rest and wait for it to pass, before restarting the exercise.

- **Leg cramps at night.** This is one of the most common and annoying symptoms I hear about from Bump Plan members, as it tends to wake them from very precious, much-needed sleep. You may also find that there's tension in your calves the next day because of it. Calf and ankle mobility exercises during the day can make a difference (such as calf raises and ankle circles), as well as generally staying active.

- **Pregnancy-related lower back pain.** As your uterus grows, taking up more space in your abdominal cavity, and your ligaments relax, this can cause changes to your joints and posture that lead to pregnancy-related lower back pain. Staying on top of your core strength and being mobile can make a difference, as this provides the core with the support it needs directly from the muscles during this time (hence this book's focus on strength).

What you need to know

From the second trimester you'll need to start considering some slight changes to the way you move your body, and which movements to prioritise. Your uterus, while potentially not showing much externally, will be continuing to grow and some positions may no longer be safe or comfortable. There are also some alterations happening within the muscles of the core that will affect how you train your abdominal muscles, which we'll discuss in a moment.

At 12 weeks, your uterus has grown to roughly the size of a large grapefruit. You can imagine it as a balloon being blown up gradually during pregnancy and, at some point, that growing balloon is going to become visible externally as a bump. If this is your first pregnancy, it may take slightly longer to 'show' than for someone who has been pregnant before: this is down to the muscle memory of your abdominal wall – essentially, the body knows what changes need to take place the second or third time around.

As mentioned above, with all the hormonal changes that are taking place, you may notice an increase in constipation as a symptom. As well as being both frustrating and uncomfortable, it's also not ideal from a pressure-management point of view (we'll discuss this in more depth on p. 174) and is particularly important to address if you have had a previous diastasis or prolapse (see pp. 167 and 257), as these can be negatively affected by repetitive increased intra-abdominal pressure (i.e. from straining to poo).

If it makes you feel any better about admitting you are constipated (because let's be honest, it can be a bit embarrassing), I was given an official 2-week extension on my final-year university dissertation due to chronic constipation (from stress). All my tutors had to be alerted (to help make the decision as to whether to grant me said extension), prompting an email explaining that they were sorry I was 'having a *hard time* of it at the moment'. It happens to us all at some point, and it might help to laugh (and ask for help) if possible.

You might also continue to feel some tenderness (and growth) in your breasts, so don't forget to invest in a good-quality sports bra. Wearing a supportive sports bra is important to protect the integrity of the ligaments around your breasts, and it's good practice to pay attention to them now, ahead of any further changes postnatally (a lactating breast can weigh up to 35 per cent more).

What happens to my abdominals during pregnancy?

This is a question I am asked so often, and it's an area of the body many mums-to-be think about above all others. It's understandable, given the value that is put on a woman's weight/appearance/looks, sadly – but please try to park any fears around what your tummy will look like post-baby and instead focus on how it functions during pregnancy.

Let's start by imagining someone with a heavily pregnant body. Imagine what it looks like from a side view – looking at the outline in profile. Where are they carrying their baby, and what area of the body do you think goes through the most change? The abdominal area? Correct.

While pregnant, the uterus (which houses the baby) grows upwards and outwards within the abdominal cavity. As the spine is essentially 'in the way' behind the uterus, the uterus pushes forwards on the abdominal wall and a 'bump' appears externally in the front of the abdomen; this can be seen from the side view from below the ribcage and above the pubic bone. Somewhat obviously, this is the area you will notice most change in during pregnancy, so some understanding of what exactly is changing can be beneficial.

As your pregnancy progresses, and your uterus gets bigger, the muscles of the core begin to stretch to allow for this growth. Remember that this a totally normal and functional part of pregnancy, and you do not need to fear (or attempt to prevent) these changes. Your transversus abdominis muscle (for more about each abdominal muscle, see pp. 45–51 in Part 1), which wraps around your core, stretches horizontally, almost like a corset being slowly loosened off. Your obliques will also lengthen vertically and diagonally as your bump grows. While we talk about the muscles lengthening to allow room for your baby, they will continue to play a role in supporting your spine and the weight of your uterus (don't worry – they don't just stop doing their job overnight).

The change that many women do seem aware of in their core is to their 'six-pack abdominals' – the rectus abdominis muscles. These two muscles run vertically down the centre of your stomach from the ribcage to the pelvis. I like to imagine them as two elastic bands running side by side. They do not connect directly to each other but instead attach to a piece of connective tissue called the linea alba.

As your bump grows, the two muscles (the two 'elastic bands') stretch vertically, but also move further away from each other, and the linea alba between them thins and stretches in response. This is called diastasis rectus abdominis (or diastasis recti or DRA) and is a perfectly normal response to pregnancy. It is thought that up to 100 per cent of women will have DRA by the time they reach their labour. To learn more about DRA, why it happens and how it changes postnatally, head to p. 167, where diastasis and prolapse expert Antony Lo gives us the lowdown.

Should I still train the abdominals? (Spoiler alert – yes!)

Now that you know what happens to your abdominal muscles during pregnancy, you need to think about how you will keep them strong and functional, while also allowing them to lengthen and stretch. There's a fine balance between overtraining your core and creating a huge amount of pressure and tension as your bump tries to grow, and maintaining enough strength there to support its weight.

The first thing to mention is that the transversus abdominis muscle is one of the main stabilisers of the core, helping to support your internal organs and stabilising the lower spine and pelvis. This is important when you know that you're about to start noticing an increasingly large mass form at the front of the pelvis! If you can maintain a functional transversus abdominis muscle, you will have more support (almost like a corset or pregnancy girdle) as your bump gets heavier, and this can help to prevent huge changes to your posture.

Another main stabiliser of the core is your pelvic floor. We often forget about this area, only really remembering it's a 'thing' if we notice it struggling to cope with the demands of the odd cough or sneeze. However, the pelvic floor plays an incredibly important role, working with the transversus abdominis muscle in stabilising the pelvis as the pregnancy bump grows.

Therefore, it's important that when training the core during pregnancy you make sure that the transversus abdominis and pelvic floor muscles are doing their jobs, and that you allow the rectus abdominis the chance to do its thing! There are so many exercises that target these muscles specifically, many of which you'll find throughout this book. They also show up during everyday movements, such as walking, dancing, swimming – so staying active in general is key here. These muscles can also be supported by maintaining good breathing technique (see p. 126 for more insight) and understanding pressure management (see p. 174).

Do I need to consider supine hypotensive syndrome now?

Supine hypotensive syndrome (also referred to as inferior vena cava compression syndrome) is caused when the uterus compresses the inferior vena cava when a pregnant woman is in a supine position (lying flat on your back), leading to decreased venous return centrally.[21] Essentially, the weight of your uterus (now that it's getting heavier) when you are lying supine, can restrict the blood flow back to your heart and symptoms can include pallor, dizziness, low blood pressure, sweating, nausea and increased heart rate. It's obviously not ideal, and given that it usually comes on after 3–10 minutes of being supine, I recommend avoiding exercises that keep you in a supine position for too long.

Now you may find you wake up lying on your back overnight, but don't panic. Chances are you are waking up *because* you're on your back, and you simply need to flip back on to your side (I know, it's not always comfortable – I'm a front sleeper!). However, it's helpful to be aware of supine hypotensive syndrome in case you happen to be in a Pilates or yoga class and the instructor sets you up in an exercise on your back – you'll need to change positions regularly to avoid feeling unwell.

There's an additional risk related to being in the supine position, as standing up from it too quickly can lower blood pressure and increase your risk of fainting, dizziness or light-headedness – this is called orthostatic hypotension. As pregnancy progresses, the volume of the circulatory system expands and blood pressure tends to fall; however, it returns to normal after delivery. Do keep this in mind when changing positions quickly during a workout.

What is the focus in weeks 13–19?

Babies are heavy. Not just once they arrive, but already now, and moving forwards (they're only going to get heavier). And it's not just the baby you're carrying; it's also the contents of your womb, including amniotic fluid, placenta, the extra blood you now have in your body (remember, there is up to 50 per cent more in pregnancy) and potentially heavier breasts. This puts a large demand through the postural chain (the muscles that run up the back of the body and keep you upright).

In the second trimester, it's important to strengthen the postural chain, so that all its muscles show up and support you, literally. These include the calves, hamstrings, glutes, erector spinae and more, and are big, powerful, important muscles.

You'll notice that in your current exercises there are some really functional postural chain ones to help keep these muscles active throughout your pregnancy. You may find that as you progress, these become more challenging, as the postural muscles get more tired due to their daily demand. That is understandable. Listen to your body and do what you can, when you can. When performing your cardiovascular (Sweat) exercises, aim to keep the intensity moderate (that's around 7/10 on the difficulty scale). Keep checking in on how hard you're working and remember, what you can do in week 13 might be different to what you can do in week 19.

Your exercises: weeks 13–19

The guidelines for activity for the second trimester are the same as the first (while considering what we've discussed so far in this chapter). You are still aiming for at least 150 minutes of moderate intensity activity per week, and to engage in muscle strengthening activity 2 days of the week.

Your warm-up and cool-down exercises can be found on pp. 74–76 and 87–88. The following exercises are all suitable as you move through the first half of the second trimester.

Strength exercises

Dumb waiters (suitable for TTC, entire pregnancy, if comfortable, and postnatal all phases)

This is one of my absolute go-to exercises, and everyone can benefit from it. The movement involves external rotation of the arm in the shoulder socket – the opposite movement to how we spend so much of our lives (hunched over laptops, hands on steering wheels, typing on our phones).

1. You can start standing or seated for this exercise, with your arms by your sides, elbows bent to 90°, palms facing upwards and hands shoulder-width apart.
2. Imagine you have a plate of spaghetti on each hand and a newspaper in each armpit.
3. Inhale to prepare and, as you exhale, start to move your hands further apart, keeping hold of both newspapers and spaghetti, until you can go no further.
4. Inhale to return to your start position.
5. Repeat.

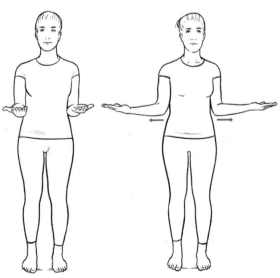

TIP: This exercise is about rotation of the arm in the shoulder socket, so make sure that everything else stays steady and stable. Your spine shouldn't be moving as your arms move – this usually signifies cheating.

REGRESSION: simply use a smaller range of movement or put actual props under the armpits and on your hands to help encourage good technique.

PROGRESSION: try holding a resistance band or loop in each hand, so that as you pull your hands apart, there is resistance, too. You could also hold a dumbbell in each hand, although this would challenge your biceps, rather than the external rotators of the arm.

Hip hinges to squats (suitable for TTC, entire pregnancy, if comfortable, and postnatal phases 1 and 2)

Following on from learning the hip hinge technique in the TTC section (do revisit that on p. 80, if needed), we now add in a knee hinge to turn this into a squat. Encouraging a hip hinge first adds a challenge for the postural chain.

1. Start in a half-hip hinge position, with feet hip-width apart, hands in prayer position and a nice, neutral spine.
2. Inhale to bend your knees, as though you're about to sit down on a chair.
3. Exhale to stand back up to your start position.
4. Repeat.

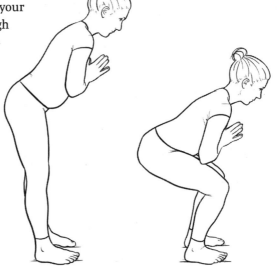

TIP: If you find your lower back takes over, is unhappy or feels very tight, try engaging your core slightly to help support the muscles of the lower back. To do this, try lifting the pelvic floor slightly, then activating your transversus abdominis muscle (like you're doing up some tight jeans).

REGRESSION: take away the half-hip hinge and go straight from standing in neutral to a squat. This is ideal for anyone who finds their lower back isn't happy during this exercise.

PROGRESSION: hold a dumbbell in each hand for extra resistance, tie a resistance band or loop around the knees to challenge the hip abductors or add a Pilates ball or yoga block between the knees to activate the hip adductors.

Side-lying leg lifts (suitable for TTC, entire pregnancy, if comfortable, and postnatal phases 1 and 2)

I love a side-lying leg lift, particularly during pregnancy, as it's a comfortable position for most people, activates the hip abductors and challenges pelvic stability.

1. Start by lying on your right-hand side, legs straight and stacked one on top of the other, with the feet slightly in front of the hips (so your body is in the shape of a banana), right arm extended along the floor, to use as a pillow for your head, and hips stacked.
2. Inhale to prepare and, as you exhale, lift the left leg as high as you can while continuing to keep your pelvis still.
3. Inhale to lower it with control.
4. Repeat on the other side.

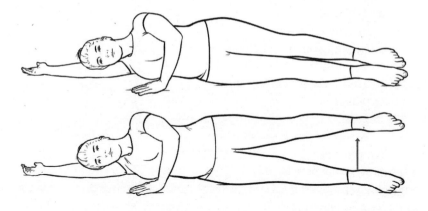

TIP: This is not a Jane Fonda workout, and you do not need to get your leg to your ear. You just take the leg as high as is comfortable, without side bending your whole body. The pelvis should stay still – it's all about the leg moving within the hip socket.

REGRESSION: reduce the range of movement or bend your bottom knee to give you more support on the floor.

PROGRESSION: tie a resistance band around your ankles to increase the resistance on the lift.

Zips (suitable for TTC, entire pregnancy, if comfortable, and postnatal all phases)

To me, zips are an absolute staple for women. They teach us how to activate the core in a way that encourages us not to bear down on the pelvic floor and are a fantastic way to strengthen it, as well as the transversus abdominis.

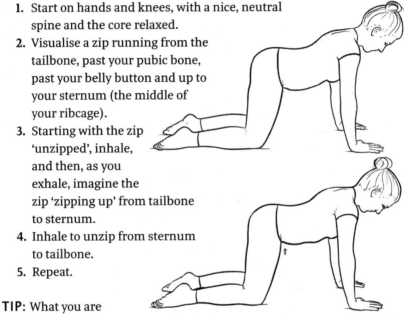

1. Start on hands and knees, with a nice, neutral spine and the core relaxed.
2. Visualise a zip running from the tailbone, past your pubic bone, past your belly button and up to your sternum (the middle of your ribcage).
3. Starting with the zip 'unzipped', inhale, and then, as you exhale, imagine the zip 'zipping up' from tailbone to sternum.
4. Inhale to unzip from sternum to tailbone.
5. Repeat.

TIP: What you are essentially doing here is engaging your pelvic floor and the transversus abdominis on the zipping up, and then releasing them on the unzip. You could also try imagining closing the anus, vagina and urethra, then drawing your tummy in as you zip up, and then releasing them in order for the unzip. When looking down at your tummy, you should be able to see some movement as you zip up (a lifting of the tummy), and on the unzip notice a release.

REGRESSION: try this in other positions, such as standing or kneeling, where you aren't having to support your weight through your arms. You could also spend time perfecting abdominal hollowing (see p. 78) first, before revisiting zips.

PROGRESSION: you could try this in a half- or full-plank position, although you may find the increased challenge makes it harder to 'feel' the zip action happening.

Side planks (suitable for TTC, entire pregnancy, if comfortable, and postnatal phase 2)

Side planks are one of those exercises that people are unsure about during pregnancy, but as long as you are managing your pressure well (see p. 174), there is no reason you can't include them in your training and they're a fantastic way of promoting oblique endurance and core strength.

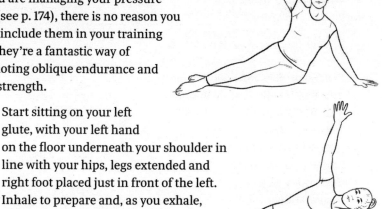

1. Start sitting on your left glute, with your left hand on the floor underneath your shoulder in line with your hips, legs extended and right foot placed just in front of the left.
2. Inhale to prepare and, as you exhale, press into your left arm and the sides of your feet, lift the hips up and aim to bring the body into a diagonal line from shoulder to feet.

TIP: This is a side plank, not a side bend, so ensure that you aim for a nice, neutral line from head to toe. Try not to sink into your supporting arm and try to keep the hips stacked, rather than allowing the pelvis to rotate.

REGRESSION: start with bent knees, and as you lift up, rest on your knees, rather than your feet. This means that your side plank is a neutral line from knees to shoulder.

PROGRESSION: stack the feet one on top of the other, so you lose some of the stability (and have to work harder); or once in your side plank, lift the top leg up towards the ceiling, so your lower leg has to work harder to keep you lifted.

Sweat exercises

Lunge kicks (suitable for TTC, entire pregnancy, if comfortable, and postnatal phase 2)

Lunges are really functional, as many of the movements we make during the day involve a lunge of some sort – walking, climbing the stairs, getting up off the floor, etc.

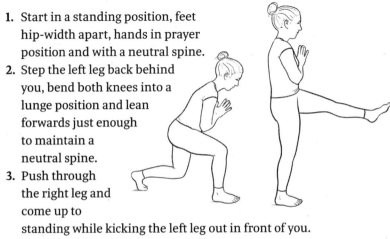

1. Start in a standing position, feet hip-width apart, hands in prayer position and with a neutral spine.
2. Step the left leg back behind you, bend both knees into a lunge position and lean forwards just enough to maintain a neutral spine.
3. Push through the right leg and come up to standing while kicking the left leg out in front of you.
4. Repeat as required, and then switch legs.

TIP: Try to encourage your standing/front leg to do the work – for example, if you're stepping your left leg back, try to push through your right leg to come to standing. Aim to keep the spine neutral as you lunge, rather than rigidly keeping your chest lifted which can cause you to back bend.

REGRESSION: this can be a wobbly exercise, so if it's too unstable, try putting your foot down on the floor to rebalance between the lunge and the kick. You could also regress it into either a lunge or a squat kick, rather than a lunge kick.

PROGRESSION: hold a dumbbell in each hand to add resistance or pick up the pace.

Crabs (suitable for TTC, entire pregnancy, if comfortable, and postnatal phases 1 and 2)

Not everyone loves squats, but there's no denying that they can be really effective at strengthening the lower body ahead of late pregnancy and labour. These 'crabs' will help develop endurance in the legs.

1. Start at the left end of your mat, in a parallel squat position, with hands in prayer position at your chest.
2. Step your left leg to the side, maintaining your squat depth, and then 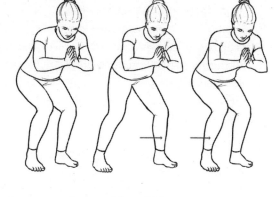 bring your right leg in, so your feet are hip-width apart.
3. Repeat, until you get to the other end of your mat, and then come back again in the same way.

TIP: Try to stay low here – you shouldn't be bouncing up and down as you move. You need to maintain a neutral spine from the side, so really think about the shape you are creating with your spine.

REGRESSION: rather than staying low, you can come up to standing between each side step, which can help to reduce some of the lactic-acid burn in the quads.

PROGRESSION: hold a dumbbell in each hand to add resistance; or tie a resistance band or loop around your knees to make it harder to abduct the legs.

Skaters (suitable for TTC, entire pregnancy, if comfortable, and postnatal phase 2)

Skaters can be adapted in so many ways to make them suitable for most stages of pregnancy, and they are one of my favourite cardiovascular moves.

1. Stand at the left end of your mat, facing the longer edge.
2. Leap towards the right end of your mat, extending your arms out wide and landing as softly as you can on your right leg, taking your left foot out behind you in mid-air, like a tail.
3. Leap to the left-hand side of your mat, landing on your left leg and taking your right foot out behind you like a tail.
4. Repeat.

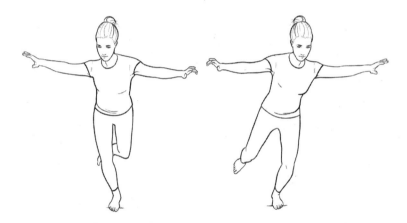

TIP: This move is designed to be quite explosive, and for you to rise up as you jump and then drop quite low when you land. This requires more work from the lower body on the recoil and managing the impact on landing.

REGRESSION: rather than leaping from side to side, you could simply side step here and remove the impact altogether. You could try smaller steps, too, or, if balance is an issue, you can put the second foot on the floor for support on landing, rather than having it behind you in mid-air.

PROGRESSION: try adding a dumbbell in each hand to add resistance as you reach the arms out on the leap; or pick up the pace.

Runner's lunges (suitable for TTC, entire pregnancy, if comfortable, and postnatal phase 2)

Runner's lunges are, perhaps obviously, a great drill for improving running technique. They can help improve your bounce (which reduces your impact when running) and are fantastic at strengthening the glutes, hamstrings and quads.

1. Stand with feet hip-width apart, arms in a running position and a neutral spine.
2. Lunge back with your right leg, bending both knees and leaning forwards slightly.
3. Push yourself back up to standing and, as you do so, bring your right knee up and through towards your chest, while jumping up from your left leg.
4. Land as softly as you can on your left foot and take your right leg back into a lunge again.
5. Repeat as required and then switch legs.

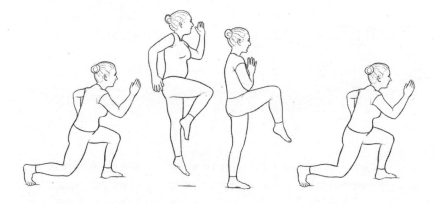

TIP: This is a very wobbly exercise, so slow it down as much as is needed, so that you can really focus on the technique. The aim is for the front/standing leg to be doing the work here and the calves to be working hard to support the jump.

REGRESSION: remove the jump. This means that you lunge, and simply come back to standing, bringing your back leg in towards the chest before repeating. Or instead of jumping off your standing leg, simply calf raise instead, so you still get your calf working, but you don't have the impact or instability to deal with.

PROGRESSION: add some dumbbells in the hands to increase resistance; or pick up the pace.

Skiing (suitable for TTC, entire pregnancy, if comfortable, and postnatal phase 2)

Skiing is a real leg burner, I'm afraid. It boosts endurance in the lower half of the body (as actual skiing would) and strengthens the calves.

1. Start in a squat position, with your legs together, feet parallel and hands in prayer position.
2. Jump up and open the legs out, so that you land in a sumo squat position, with your feet wider than hip-width apart and in turnout.
3. Jump up and land with your legs together again in your start position.
4. Repeat.

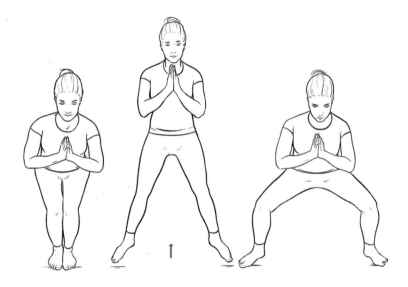

TIP: This exercise is designed to be very bouncy, but try to land as softly as you can (this makes it harder but reduces the impact). Aim to maintain a neutral spine as you move – think about the shapes you're creating with your body.

REGRESSION: instead of jumping into each squat position, you can step out and in, therefore removing the impact altogether.

PROGRESSION: add a dumbbell in each hand; or pick up the pace.

Example routines

Below, you'll find two example routines. Routine 1 combines all of the exercise options. Routine 2 combines all of the Sweat exercises with a rest period (which you do not have to utilise). Feel free to repeat the routines to help you build up to the recommended 150 minutes of physical activity per week (an example week could be 5 x 30 minute workouts).

Routine 1

- *Warm-up*
- Lunge kicks: 30–60 seconds
- Dumb waiters: 30–60 seconds
- Crabs: 30–60 seconds
- Hip hinges to squats: 30–60 seconds
- Skaters: 30–60 seconds
- Side-lying leg lifts: 30–60 seconds
- Runner's lunges: 30–60 seconds
- Zips: 30–60 seconds
- Skiing: 30–60 seconds
- Side planks: 30–60 seconds
- *Repeat or cool-down* (if repeating, don't exceed four sets and be sure to include a rest period if you need it between sets)

Routine 2

- *Warm-up*
- Lunge kicks: 30–60 seconds
- Rest – marching on the spot: 60 seconds
- Crabs: 30–60 seconds

- Rest – marching on the spot: 60 seconds
- Skaters: 30–60 seconds
- Rest – marching on the spot: 60 seconds
- Runner's lunges: 30–60 seconds
- Rest – marching on the spot: 60 seconds
- Skiing: 30–60 seconds
- *Repeat or cool-down* (if repeating, don't exceed four sets and be sure to include a rest period if you need it between sets)

Your pelvic floor exercise

Sucking through a straw

This is another really helpful visualisation to encourage good technique. It teaches the concept of both a squeeze and a lift, which is what you want when practising your pelvic floor exercises.

1. Start in a comfortable position – this might be seated, lying, side-lying, standing.
2. Close your eyes (this will help you to focus internally) and try to clear your mind.
3. Focus on your breathing by bringing your awareness to breathing in and out through your nose. Relax your jaw and ensure your tongue is relaxed in your mouth.
4. Imagine you have a straw placed inside the vagina: inhale and, as you exhale, imagine sucking a thick smoothie up through the straw.
5. Inhale to release and allow the smoothie to slowly fall back out of the straw.
6. Repeat 8–10 times.

TIP: I want you to imagine that the smoothie is *really* thick (you know, one of those that's ridiculously healthy but looks and tastes like pondweed). As you exhale, think about the drawing up and in (squeezing and lifting) that would be required to actually suck the smoothie up. When you release, let the smoothie fall back down the straw (not firing it out, though). If you find this visualisation too weird, feel free to imagine sucking a tampon up inside you instead.

Mind the gap: understanding diastasis

by Antony Lo, musculoskeletal physiotherapist

Diastasis rectus abdominis (DRA – also known as diastasis recti (DR) among other names) is a condition where the tissue between your two rectus abdominis muscles – the linea alba – is stretched but not torn. This leads to the appearance of a 'gap' between your 'six-pack' muscles. This can happen to men and children, but is most commonly seen in women – especially those who have been pregnant. Diastasis is *not* about the skin and the fat between the skin and the muscles – these can become stretched there and be aesthetically displeasing for the person concerned, but it does not mean they have a DRA.

Diastasis is very common in the pregnant and postnatal population. Around 67–100 per cent of pregnant women will have diastasis of some form during their pregnancy. After giving birth (whether vaginally or via Caesarean section), around 40 per cent will have a diastasis at about 8 weeks and about 33 per cent at 12 months. About 50 per cent of people under the age of 45 and about 23–25 per cent in both the 45–60 and the 60-plus age groups have a diastasis.

The major contributing factor to developing DRA is pregnancy and the growing baby/babies inside the uterus. However, obesity, especially in those with higher abdominal visceral fat (fat around the organs in the abdomen) and diabetes (including gestational diabetes) are also contributing factors. Other risk factors like hypermobility, exercise, age and size during pregnancy do exist, but don't have particularly strong evidence behind them.

Claims of how you can 'cure' or 'fix' your diastasis appear to be a favourite topic on social media. But at the time of writing, there is simply no proven way to prevent it, nor is there any proven, non-surgical way of improving the aesthetics or the 'gap' between the muscles. However, we do know that natural recovery happens for most people – up to two in every three at 12 months postpartum.

In the absence of strong evidence of any one particular way to help prevent and manage DRA, understanding the principles behind the main concerns about it becomes very important. One key principle is to get stronger – because this helps to develop resilience and prepares people for the awkward lifting and twisting that are a part of normal parenting life. Another key principle is to ensure that you challenge the linea alba and other tissues because that's what's going to strengthen them. However, excessive tension – and too little – may not be helpful. But the good news is that it is unlikely most people create excessive amounts of pressure during activities – more on this a bit later.

Health and fitness professionals are mainly concerned about people with diastasis developing conditions like abdominal hernias, pelvic floor dysfunction (like urinary and faecal incontinence), pelvic organ prolapse and conditions such as back pain and other issues. Hernias develop when excessive tension causes a tear or a split in the abdominal muscles and/or fascia. But we know tissue needs *some* tension to adapt. To get a sense of how much tension is the right amount, it's helpful to understand the concepts of 'hard doming' and 'soft doming'. 'Doming' is where the tummy might bulge out a bit (into a dome or cone or tent-type shape). People are usually advised to avoid 'doming' altogether, but the fear surrounding if you are 'doming' or not is not worth such strict recommendations. Instead, I suggest you test yourself or have someone test you for soft doming. If you can exercise and the midline of your abdomen is level with your ribs and pelvic bones *and* the tension feels soft or squashy to the touch, then it is unlikely that you're experiencing hard enough doming to develop a hernia.

Pelvic issues such as incontinence (leaking) and pelvic organ prolapse are thought to be due to excessive amounts of pressure within the abdomen pushing down into the pelvic cavity and especially the vagina. If you have a diastasis, it might be your body's way of managing the pressure on the pelvic floor. In fact, there are hints in the research that having a diastasis might even be helpful in the early postpartum period to decrease the pressure and the possible risk of developing pelvic organ prolapse.

Bearing all of these factors in mind when exercising, it is important to remember that the World Health Organization and health organisations around the world recommend that postpartum people achieve 150 minutes of moderate intensity exercise per week, including at least two sessions of whole-body strengthening *and* pelvic floor exercises for people during pregnancy and postpartum. Therefore, *how* you exercise is more important than the exercise you choose. Whatever you're doing, keep the tension in the midline relatively soft. In any case, the whole-health benefits of exercise far outweigh the concerns about diastasis. Therefore, keep exercising in ways that you want to.

If, after 2–3 years postnatally, you still have a diastasis of 5cm or more, and it concerns you aesthetically, you might consider an abdominoplasty. However, this may be difficult before 2 years postpartum if you don't have a good support network to assist you in caring for your child. It is a major abdominal operation from which proper recovery will take months, so consult your healthcare provider about the right way to manage it for you.

To summarise:

- Diastasis is very common – most women will have it in late pregnancy and around one in three will have it at 12 months postpartum.
- There's not much you can do to prevent it. Moderate levels of activity and exercises might help improve it (unproven by research). Being mindful of soft vs hard doming might be helpful to calm the fears of developing a hernia, pain or pelvic floor dysfunction.
- Treat any claims made by people about being able to 'cure' your diastasis with caution because there are no proven, non-surgical ways to prevent or improve it.
- Observe the physical activity recommendations for pregnant and postpartum people – 150 minutes of moderate intensity exercise, including two sessions of whole-body strengthening.
- Surgery may be needed, especially for aesthetic reasons, but there is a lot of guidance and exercises that can be used in the meantime which may be helpful.

Pregnancy weeks 20–27

We are at the halfway point, people! Well, in theory, anyway. Maybe you're thinking, Only halfway . . . how? Or maybe it has totally flown by. Second time around for me it really has been whizzing by (maybe writing this book has helped with that), and I'll be honest, there have been times where I have lost count of how many weeks I am.

This is the stage where – hopefully – some of the toughest pregnancy symptoms from the first 20 weeks start to ease, and people do tend to speak about feeling a little more 'normal'. I really hope for everyone that is the case, but if not, I'm thinking of you and sending strength.

Your baby is about to have a big growth spurt, and you'll also start to feel them move during this period, which can be so magical . . . until, that is, they decide that bedtime is party time and sleep gets even harder to come by (we'll let them off, though).

If you are UK-based, you'll likely have an anomaly scan around 20 weeks and some of you may choose to find out the sex of your baby at this appointment. We chose not to find out for both babies, and to have a lovely surprise (although I don't remember the point in labour when I found out Freya was a girl), but I can also see how much easier it would be to know from both a bonding and an organisational point of view.

Your body

As mentioned, you are now, hopefully, noticing a slight decline in some of the miserable pregnancy symptoms that can come in the first half; however, there are some new ones that can creep in as your body starts to really develop a bump. Remember that the whole body takes the strain of a growing uterus, not just the abdominals, so it's understandable that you may start to feel aches or pains in other areas.

Here are a few of the most common symptoms you may experience at this stage:

- **Sleeping problems.** Sleeping on your side becomes the only option available, and if that is not your normal sleeping position, it can feel so unnatural. Try lying with a pillow under your bump, knees bent and a pillow between your knees.
- **Haemorrhoids.** These are swellings around or inside your anus, containing enlarged blood vessels. They can happen to anyone, but are more common during pregnancy due to the hormonal changes to your veins, and especially if you suffer with constipation.
- **Stretch marks.** These are very common (it's thought eight in ten pregnant women develop stretch marks during pregnancy). There is no solid evidence that creams work to prevent or reduce stretch marks, but you may find they ease the itchiness that can come with them.

- **Rib pain.** As the uterus grows, it moves up towards the ribcage. Around now, you might be starting to notice it's a little harder to breathe deeply (I recommend practising the breathwork described on p. 126 to help with this) and that your ribcage is getting wider. As the ribs are pushed outwards (and some of you develop a bit of 'rib flare'), you may experience pain or discomfort. Postnatally, we will be addressing this change in the ribcage and aiming to bring them back to some sort of normal.
- **Braxton Hicks.** Sometimes called practice contractions or false labour pains, these are caused by the contracting and relaxing of the womb and are totally harmless. They are irregular and don't build in intensity, which distinguishes them from 'real' contractions. They can be brought on during physical activity (and sex, actually), so if you notice them while exercising, do feel free to pause until they have passed, and then carry on, if you wish.

What you need to know

By now, you'll no doubt have a noticeable bump – your baby is around 26cm tall, after all – and your uterus will be taking up a fair portion of your abdominal cavity. As this happens, pressure is placed on your linea alba (the tissue that runs between the two rectus abdominis muscles) and down into the pelvic floor. It can really help to understand the concept of 'pressure management', so that you manage the increased pressure well while exercising and give your core the support it needs at this time.

What on earth is pressure management?

I want you to visualise the abdominal cavity, which is the space between the diaphragm (see pp. 124–125) and the pelvic floor (see pp. 51–55). The abdominal cavity is a hollow space filled with fluid, organs (such as the stomach, kidneys, intestines), muscles (such as the abdominals) and part of your spine. These all create a certain amount of pressure inside the abdominal cavity (called intra-abdominal pressure) that pushes outwards on the front, sides, base and back of the trunk.

Now try to imagine the abdominal cavity as a balloon. When you blow up a balloon, the air inside exerts pressure outwards in

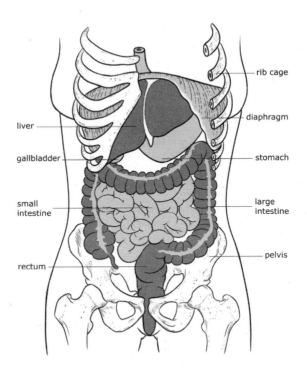

liver

gallbladder

small
intestine

rectum

rib cage

diaphragm

stomach

large
intestine

pelvis

all directions, giving it its shape; this air is the equivalent of all the 'stuff' in your abdominal cavity. When you squeeze a balloon (that has been blown up and knotted), you increase the pressure within it, and the air inside doesn't escape, but is pushed to other parts of the balloon in response. Usually, the pressure is pushed equally to other areas, and the whole balloon changes shape, until it is released again.

Coming back to you: when you move your body, cough, sneeze, poo, you activate muscles within the core which squeeze it (like the balloon being squeezed) and increase the intra-abdominal pressure. Rather than everything in the abdominal cavity being squeezed out, in an ideal world, the pressure is redistributed to the rest of core.

However, during pregnancy things can change slightly. You can start to develop 'paths of least resistance' in your linea alba and pelvic floor. Previously, we discussed the fact that a growing bump causes a thinning and widening of the linea alba, and can also weaken the pelvic floor. During pregnancy, what can happen is that when pressure is created in the core, it is forced towards the path of least resistance, rather than the entire core. So you might notice a lot of doming or coning down the middle of your bump (where pressure is pushing at the linea alba) or feel lots of bearing down on your pelvic floor (or leaking, due to the pressure being too great to handle).

Ultimately, pregnancy can make it more challenging to manage the pressure, which isn't ideal.

What does this mean for me?

While you want to make sure you challenge your core muscles and keep them working and stimulated, you also need to make sure you're not creating so much pressure in the core that you can't manage it. If you notice lots of hard doming (where your tummy goes very pointy down the midline and feels uncomfortable and hard when touched) or you are leaking during an exercise, you should consider whether that movement is helping or hindering you. It might be that you need to regress the exercise in question (make it easier) or avoid it altogether.

For one person this might mean they can no longer do a full-plank at 20 weeks, as it may leave them with hard doming down their midline, and become too challenging for them to manage that pressure. Well, that's fine, and the solution is to swap to a half-plank and see how that feels. However, someone else might manage a full-plank at 20 weeks perfectly fine (for transparency, I couldn't do one at 20 weeks without doming) and continue to practise them until 26 weeks. The same goes for crunches or sit-ups – if they're uncomfortable or you experience doming, either regress the movement or try an alternative.

We are all different, and what is important here is that you focus on how each movement feels for *you*. As previously mentioned, all your listed exercises have regressions and progressions, so use these to ensure that the moves work for you.

What is the focus in weeks 20–27?

Taking all I've said into account, you do still want a strong, functional core, and avoiding all abdominal work is not a good plan. We often forget, though, that muscles rarely work in isolation – they work as a team – and lots of the exercises in The Bump Plan stimulate the core and play a huge role in keeping it functioning, even though they might not feel like specific abdominal exercises.

The same is also true of the pelvic floor muscles: they're often recruited during exercises that target the lower body and in a very functional way. Remember that you won't only ever need your pelvic floor muscles while you're sitting cross-legged, thinking about your breath – you'll also need them while lunging to stop your toddler falling over or when you run to catch a bus. So we'll be strengthening them, too, in these exercises (particularly the Sweat ones), don't you worry!

Your exercises: weeks 20–27

Your warm-up and cool-down exercises can be found on pp. 74–76 and 87–88. Now let's take a look at your exercises for the second half of your second trimester.

Strength exercises

Banded breathwork (suitable for TTC, entire pregnancy, if comfortable, and postnatal, all phases)

This is a great way to strengthen the diaphragm muscle (our primary breathing muscle), which is often forgotten. At this stage of pregnancy, the growing uterus makes the diaphragm's job a little more difficult, so it's important to show it some love.

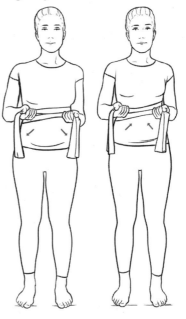

1. This can be performed standing or seated. Wrap a resistance band, scarf or dressing-gown belt gently around the back of the ribcage and bring it round to the front, holding it there, crossed over.
2. As you inhale, imagine breathing into the band, causing it to slightly tighten around the ribcage, as the ribcage expands in all directions.
3. As you exhale, you should feel the band release and slacken back off.

TIP: This is about encouraging the ribcage to move as you breathe, which helps the diaphragm muscle to do its job. Try to imagine the ribcage expanding in a 360° fashion as you inhale, and then draw back inwards on the exhale.

REGRESSION: don't worry if you don't have a prop to tie around the ribcage; you can simply rest your hands on the sides (or front and back) of the ribcage to gain feedback as you breathe.

PROGRESSION: there are no real progressions of this exercise, as what is most important is nailing the technique, and repetition.

Elevated knee lifts (suitable for TTC, entire pregnancy, if comfortable, and postnatal phases 1 and 2)

This is a great way to challenge the abdominals, while having a great view of the core and assessing how well you are managing pressure there (see p. 174 for more on pressure management).

1. Start seated on the floor, resting back on your forearms, with your knees bent and feet on the floor, hip-width apart, and a neutral spine.
2. Inhale and then, as you exhale, lift your right leg up to a tabletop position.
3. Inhale to release it back to the floor.
4. Exhale to lift the left leg up to tabletop.
5. Inhale to release.

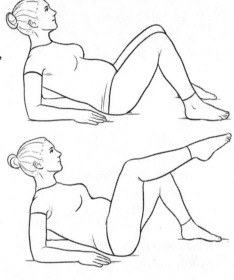

TIP: This exercise is all about stability, so as you move/lift your leg, try not to move the spine or pelvis as well – they should stay stable.

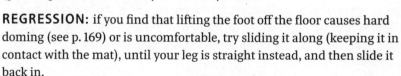

REGRESSION: if you find that lifting the foot off the floor causes hard doming (see p. 169) or is uncomfortable, try sliding it along (keeping it in contact with the mat), until your leg is straight instead, and then slide it back in.

PROGRESSION: try lifting the leg to tabletop and then extending it out on the diagonal as low as you can manage the pressure, before bringing it back to tabletop and then lowering it back to the floor.

Arm reaches (suitable for TTC, entire pregnancy, if comfortable, and postnatal, all phases)

We spend so much of our lives with our arms reaching down and in front of us, particularly once we have children, so it's important we balance this out with shoulder flexion. This looks simple but can be really challenging.

1. Start on hands and knees, with a neutral spine, knees hip-width apart and hands shoulder-width apart.
2. Inhale to prepare and then, as you exhale, without moving your spine, reach your right arm up and forwards, bringing it as high as you can maintaining a neutral spine.
3. Inhale to release it back to the floor.
4. Exhale to repeat with the left arm.

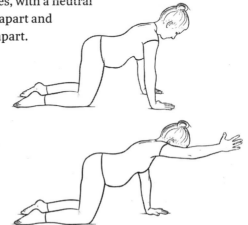

TIP: This exercise is about getting your arm to move within the shoulder socket, which is why it's important to keep the rest of the body still and stable. Activating your core, or imagining hugging your ribcage in slightly, could help you to get the arm higher without compromising your neutral spine.

REGRESSION: you could first try this seated or standing, so there is no need to weight bear on your other arm and you can focus on the moving arm alone.

PROGRESSION: try holding a dumbbell in the hand you are lifting to add resistance; or try kneeling on one end of a resistance band and holding the other end in the hand you are lifting, again for extra resistance.

Thoracic extensions (suitable for TTC, entire pregnancy, if comfortable, and postnatal, all phases)

We all need more thoracic extension in our lives, and it usually feels amazing. We spend a lot of time looking down, and so taking the opportunity to look up and extend our upper backs is really important.

1. This can be done standing, seated or kneeling. Ensure you start with a neutral spine, hands by your temples and elbows wide.

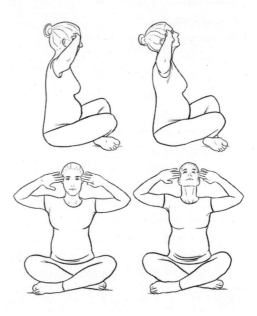

2. As you inhale, start to take your eyeline up towards the ceiling, lifting the chest upwards and extending your upper back (your thoracic spine).

3. As you exhale, slowly lower your gaze, and your chest, back to your neutral start position.

TIP: This is about thoracic extension – it is not a big back bend, and it's not a case of simply pulling your head back and looking at the ceiling. When in extension, the back of your neck should be smooth, not wrinkly, and it's about lifting the chest up, rather than back.

REGRESSION: remove the arms from the equation, as they can make the exercise harder; instead, allow them to rest in your lap or have them crossed over your chest.

PROGRESSION: reach your arms up overhead (by your ears) and take them with you as you extend the spine; or interlace your fingers and put your hands behind your head to deepen the stretch across the chest during extension.

Palm ups (suitable for TTC, entire pregnancy, if comfortable, and postnatal, all phases)

Similar to dumb waiters, these encourage the arm to move in the shoulder socket, in a way it doesn't do enough during modern-day life. We are focusing on external rotation of the arm here, which can feel hard, but is so important.

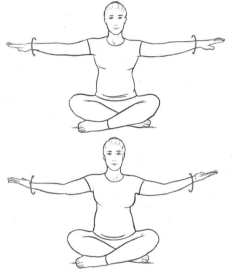

1. Either seated, standing or kneeling, start with a neutral spine, arms extended out to your sides and palms facing the floor, elbows soft.
2. On your exhale, rotate your arms, so that the palms now face the ceiling, then rotate and turn the palms down again.
3. Start to pick up the pace – this should be quite a fast movement.

TIP: While you are turning the palms to face both down *and* up here, focus on the turning up. Really try to get your little finger as high as possible, to get as much external rotation as you can at the shoulder.

REGRESSION: if you bend your elbow more, you may find you feel slightly more rotation at the shoulder, and your arms ache less (although that burn you feel in the shoulder is what you are after).

PROGRESSION: add dumbbells in the hands for extra resistance to a group of triangular shoulder muscles called the deltoids.

Sweat exercises

Split punches (suitable for TTC, entire pregnancy, if comfortable, and postnatal phase 2)

Split punches are a fun, bouncy cardiovascular exercise and one of my absolute favourites! Don't forget your sports bra, though.

1. Stand with feet hip-width apart, right leg out slightly in front and left arm in front in a punching position.

2. Jump up and swap over, so that the left leg is out in front and the right arm is punching forwards.
3. Repeat.

TIP: It's important you have the opposite arm and opposite leg out in front of you here, otherwise it can feel very strange. Try to land as softly as you can (this is harder) and keep the spine upright in neutral.

REGRESSION: the low-impact option here would be to step one foot forwards (as well as punching with the opposite arm) and then bring the foot and arm back in, then step the other foot forwards and punch with the opposite arm – essentially, removing the jump and simply stepping a foot forwards. You could also slow the move down.

PROGRESSION: add a dumbbell in each hand; or pick up the pace.

Knee pulls (suitable for TTC, entire pregnancy, if comfortable, and postnatal phase 2)

This exercise is great not only for getting your heart rate up, but also for challenging your hip stability (especially as you're standing on a single leg). I love the burn on this.

1. Stand with your feet hip-width apart.
2. Bend your knees into a mini squat, hip hinge slightly, take your right leg out behind you (keeping the right foot lightly touching the floor) and reach your arms overhead by your ears.

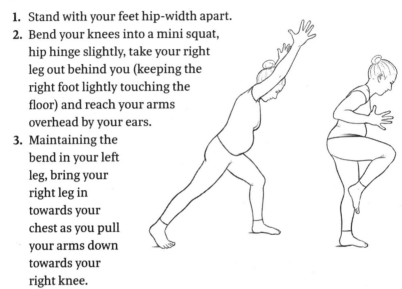

3. Maintaining the bend in your left leg, bring your right leg in towards your chest as you pull your arms down towards your right knee.
4. Open back out to your start position and repeat on the other side.

TIP: You are trying to keep the standing knee bent here, so there should be no bobbing up and down as you move. Try to keep your pelvis level (not dropping to one side) and keep the weight on your standing leg – your back leg should only really kiss the floor, rather than support your weight.

REGRESSION: for some, this exercise may be too much of a challenge for the lower back. If it's unhappy, you could either just do the leg movement here and have your arms in prayer position or just the arm movement, keeping your back foot in contact with the floor, rather than both leg and arm movements together.

PROGRESSION: hold a dumbbell in each hand; or imagine that you are pulling on resistance bands as you pull the arms down.

Jacks (suitable for TTC, entire pregnancy, if comfortable, and postnatal phase 2)

Jumping jacks are a staple when it comes to cardiovascular exercise and most of us will have practised them before. I give a low-impact option here, too, for those who find the impact mixed with open legs a little too much for the pelvic floor.

1. Stand with arms by your sides, elbows soft, palms facing forwards, feet together.
2. Jump up and land with the feet hip-width apart and arms overhead, before jumping back to your start position.
3. Repeat.

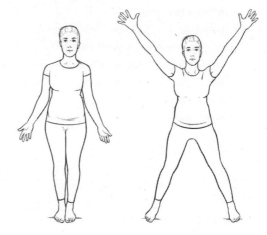

TIP: This exercise is meant to be bouncy and fast but do try to land as gently as you can (which is harder). Try not to lean backwards, which I frequently see, as this can make it harder for your abdominals to support you.

REGRESSION: if you find that you'd prefer a lower impact option, try tapping one foot out to the side as you take both arms overhead, then bringing the leg in as the arms come down. Then take the other leg out to the side and tap the floor as the arms go overhead, then bring it all back in. So it's essentially both arms and one leg, rather than both arms and both legs.

PROGRESSION: pick up the pace; or hold a dumbbell in each hand to add resistance.

Arm pulls (suitable for TTC, entire pregnancy, if comfortable, and postnatal phase 2)

We spend so much of our time hunched over in modern-day life, so any exercise that opens up the chest and works the upper back is a winner in my eyes – and this one feels great!

1. Stand with your arms stretched out in front of you, feet wider than hip-width apart.
2. Bend your right knee, bringing your foot towards your bum and shifting your weight to your left leg, while pulling the elbows backwards at shoulder height (rowing) and squeezing gently between the shoulder blades.
3. Put your right foot back down and reach the arms forwards.
4. Repeat with the left leg and the arms.

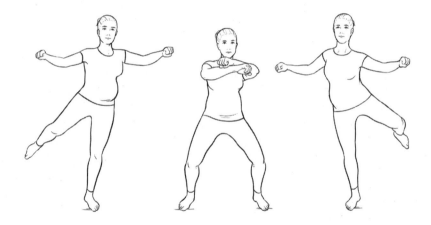

TIP: Think about the shoulder blades moving, so you really activate the mid traps and rhomboids (two of the muscle groups between the shoulders). Try to keep the spine relatively neutral, rather than body popping and shoving the ribcage forwards as you pull the arms back.

REGRESSION: slow the move down or just choose to do either the leg element (kicking the heel towards the bum) or the arm section (rowing).

PROGRESSION: you could hold a dumbbell in each hand; or hold a resistance band in your hands for the rowing element.

Skipping (suitable for TTC, entire pregnancy, if comfortable, and postnatal phase 2)

While you may feel a bit silly doing this exercise, using a pretend skipping rope (i.e. your imagination) probably makes more sense than using a real one (no broken lamps) and might also be a little safer if you aren't a regular skipper.

1. Stand, hands out by your sides, as if you are holding a skipping rope.
2. Imagine you are skipping, jumping with your legs together, and circle the arms while jumping.

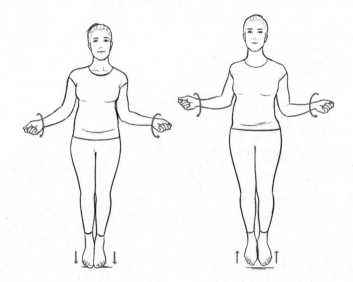

TIP: If you are performing the full exercise (rather than the low-impact version, below), try to land as softly and as bouncy as you can – this will challenge the calves more.

REGRESSION: if you prefer a lower impact option (as I do when heavily pregnant), you can simply toe tap: circle the arms as if skipping, but tap one foot out in front of you, then the other, rather than jumping.

PROGRESSION: you can hold dumbbells in each hand; or take your arms further away from your body (so they are straighter and heavier).

Example routines

Below, you'll find two example routines. Routine 1 combines all of the exercise options. Routine 2 combines all of the Sweat exercises with a rest period (which you do not have to utilise). Feel free to repeat the routines to help you build up to the recommended 150 minutes of physical activity per week (an example week could be 5 x 30 minute workouts).

Routine 1

- *Warm-up*
- Split punches: 30–60 seconds
- Banded breathwork: 30–60 seconds
- Knee pulls: 30–60 seconds
- Elevated knee lifts: 30–60 seconds
- Jacks: 30–60 seconds
- Arm extensions: 30–60 seconds
- Arm pulls: 30–60 seconds
- Thoracic extensions: 30–60 seconds
- Skipping: 30–60 seconds
- Palm ups: 30–60 seconds
- *Repeat or cool-down* (if repeating, don't exceed four sets and be sure to include a rest period if you need it between sets)

Routine 2

- *Warm-up*
- Split punches: 30–60 seconds
- Rest – marching on the spot: 60 seconds
- Knee pulls: 30–60 seconds
- Rest – marching on the spot: 60 seconds
- Jacks: 30–60 seconds

- Rest – marching on the spot: 60 seconds
- Arm pulls: 30–60 seconds
- Rest – marching on the spot: 60 seconds
- Skipping: 30–60 seconds
- *Repeat or cool-down* (if repeating, don't exceed four sets and be sure to include a rest period if you need it between sets)

Your pelvic floor exercise

Bracing check

This exercise is a test of how your pelvic floor is coping with pressure and can be really instructive. You'll be engaging the pelvic floor, creating a pressure challenge by coughing and then seeing whether the pelvic floor is still engaged or has turned off/released. Practising this could help you to cope with the demand placed on the pelvic floor when you do *actually* cough when going about your day-to-day business (as opposed to sitting still, concentrating on it).

1. Start in a comfortable position – this might be seated, lying, side-lying, standing.
2. Close your eyes (this will help you to focus internally) and try to clear your mind.
3. Focus on your breathing by bringing your awareness to breathing in and out through your nose. Relax your jaw and ensure your tongue is relaxed in your mouth.
4. Inhale and, as you exhale, squeeze and lift the pelvic floor. Hold this, and then perform a little cough. Is the pelvic floor still engaged or has it released itself?
5. Try again 5 times. The aim here is to try to maintain your pelvic floor hold, while performing your cough.

TIP: Don't panic if you struggle to keep the pelvic floor active during your cough, especially at this stage of pregnancy. You may find, though, that practising this technique helps to reduce your chance of leaking when you cough. Ensure that at the end of this exercise (when you've performed all the reps), you relax the pelvic floor by taking a few long breaths.

Understanding your mental health during the pregnancy and postnatal period

by Dr Rebecca Moore, consultant perinatal psychiatrist

Our hormones alter a lot during pregnancy, particularly oestrogen and progesterone. These changes are important for a healthy pregnancy but can also be linked to unwanted feelings, such as tiredness, sickness and mood swings.

We all come to pregnancy with our own histories and stories, and it is a huge physical and emotional transition that can often bring with it feelings of anxiety, worry, low mood or anger and rage. Many women and birthing people begin to think about how they will parent, perhaps reflect more on their own childhoods or worry about decisions needing to be made around finances or work. And, of course, partners can have all these feelings, too.

Pregnancy is a time when virtually everyone has some big feelings and mood changes at times, and day to day, there are lots of things that can help – whether trying to get plenty of sleep, if possible, or just resting more, having a good cry over a weepy film, gentle exercise you enjoy and doing the things that bring you joy, be that reading, singing, dancing or shopping. Whatever makes you feel good.

If you feel able, talking through things with your partner, friends or family can really help to explore how you are feeling; and if you can't speak it, try writing it down in a diary or journal.

Your midwife can also help, as can peer-support phone lines (such as PANDAS in the UK), which are free and offer compassionate advice from mums who understand.

Making connections with other pregnant women locally can also be a great way to share experiences. This might be via a local pregnancy yoga class, an app such as Peanut or Mush or joining a local antenatal class. Once we share, we often realise that everyone around us is having the same feelings and that can really help us feel less alone.

We all have the odd day when nothing goes right or we feel tired or tearful in pregnancy, but if it's more a case of feeling low or anxious most days, and it's a consistent change, there are lots of places you can find support. For some, pregnancy is the first time they feel low or anxious. It might be that you feel your eating has changed or your sleep, or you can't focus at work or don't want to see friends.

Your GP or midwife can often be a good place to start a conversation, and there are all kinds of things that can be added in to support you, if needed – extra midwifery visits, therapy and/or medication in some instances.

Postnatally is also, for most women, another time when mental health can change. Sleep deprivation has a big role to play for most, alongside changing hormones again and starting a feeding journey with your baby.

Almost everyone has a few days of the baby blues in the first week of being a mum, when they feel teary, restless, irritable or just a bit overwhelmed. This usually settles with no treatment needed and is not an illness.

- Around one in five women experiences a mental health change during pregnancy or within the early postnatal years; many other women will be having these experiences – you are not alone.[22]

- Studies estimate at least 50 per cent of women will hide or underplay their feelings and women are often concerned not to be perceived to be bad mums.[23]

Postnatal depression often presents with feeling low all the time, feeling there is no joy in life or not wanting to get dressed, eat or see anyone. New mums can doubt themselves, feel very anxious about parenting or even have thoughts of wanting to harm themselves.

Whatever you are feeling during pregnancy or afterwards, please know that there are lots of ways to seek support with a healthcare professional, a phone line, online in a forum or you can self-refer for therapy and support via your local Talking Therapies programme.[24] People are there to help and support you not to judge.

Let's all make maternal mental health our business, not only asking new mums to reach out, but reaching back ourselves to check in with friends, colleagues and family members who are pregnant or new mums. Making space, asking 'How are you?' and sitting and really listening can sometimes be the first part of a conversation that feels so important. We can all play a part in making pregnancy and postpartum better for all.

Resources:

Maternal Mental Health Alliance
Maternalmentalhealthalliance.org
Best Beginnings Bestbeginnings.org.uk
Make Birth Better Makebirthbetter.org
PANDAS Pandasfoundation.org.uk
Samaritans Samaritans.org
Association of Postnatal Illness Apni.org

Pregnancy weeks 28–33

~~~~~~

Week 28 marks the start of your third trimester. During this period, your baby will do lots of growing, kicking and wriggling, preparing itself for life on the outside. You might already be experiencing those rib kicks and elbow jabs to the bladder. And your emotions will no doubt range from excited, to anxious, to apprehensive, to all the above. But staying active in this last trimester will give you focus and help boost your mood.

Your body

There's no denying that the third trimester can start to feel a little challenging and/or uncomfortable at times. Your bump will be getting heavy now, given that at 28 weeks your baby already weighs around 1kg (and that's not including their baggage), but any core work you've done previously will be supporting you and absolutely paying off.

Here are some of the most common pregnancy symptoms at this stage:

- **Increased tiredness.** Yep, we're back there again. Reminiscent of that first trimester, you may feel that you need to rest more, nap more or simply sit on the sofa and stare into space more. Not always easy, I know, especially if you have other children at home, but do try to surrender to it if possible and get some extra rest in.
- **Backache.** Now, hopefully, you've been following your Bump Plan workouts for a while, and the possibility of backache is slim, but it can hit anyone at any point. Pain is multi-faceted, and can have many causes, but at this stage, backache can be caused by the relaxation of joints, the increase in weight of your bump and a change in how you move your body.
- **Carpal-tunnel syndrome.** This is an issue that can crop up at any time in life but is much more common during pregnancy and can make certain movements and positions painful. It's caused by compression of the nerves that run through the wrist, and can cause weakness, tingling, pain and numbness in the hand or arm.
- **Varicose veins and vulvar varicosities.** Varicose veins are enlarged, swollen veins and can be more common during pregnancy due to the relaxation of the walls of blood vessels and the increased volume of blood in the body. Some women may also find varicose veins on their vulva due to the increased blood flow to the pelvis.
- **Strange or disturbing dreams.** While it's not clear what causes these dreams, it's possible that they are a hormonal response, or down to the underlying emotions that can come with the changes presented by pregnancy.

What you need to know

As with the move from the first trimester to the second, there are no sweeping changes in how you should move your body when transitioning from the second to the third. You still want to aim for the recommended 'at least 150 minutes of moderate intensity physical activity per week' set out in the CMOs' guidelines, and make sure that you are combining cardiovascular training and muscle strengthening exercises to stay functionally fit.

What you might find, though, is that certain positions or movements are starting to become uncomfortable or just too challenging. This is totally understandable as your body adapts and changes to make space for your baby, and so you need to be kind to yourself and flexible with your physical activity choices.

There are almost always alterations that can be made to your training to ensure it stays comfortable, and what is most important is that you enjoy moving your body rather than dreading it. Here are a few suggestions for some of the most common issues that can creep in around this stage of pregnancy.

I'm struggling with wrist pain

Pain and sensitivity around the wrists can be quite common during pregnancy and can range from low-level pain to full-blown carpal-tunnel syndrome. The latter is caused by a swelling of the carpal tunnel (the space in the wrist that the nerves pass through), which then presses on the nerves, leading to pain, weakness and/or numbness.

Positions in which you weight-bear on your hands – such as on hands and knees, in half- or full-planks, etc. – can feel uncomfortable when you suffer with wrist pain, and so it's worth finding alternatives. There's no need to push through the pain, so here are my top suggestions:

- Try sending your weight backwards into your legs more and take some of the weight out of the arms (you don't need to have your shoulders directly above your wrists). This will also have the effect of reducing the extension of the wrist, which should make it feel more bearable.
- You can try making your hands into fists, with nice straight/ neutral wrists, and rest on these instead of your palms. That way, your wrists are in neutral and usually more comfortable.
- You can come down on to your forearms instead. This might not work for all exercises (for example, where you need to move your arms) and some people find it feels weird for their bumps, but it's an option.
- Try holding some dumbbells in your hands, resting them on the floor. This will allow you to keep your wrists straight/ neutral and lift you slightly away from the floor.

Do play around with these options and see which work best for you. Spending time in prone (on hands and knees, facing the floor) can be a great way to help get your baby into a good position for birth (which we'll discuss in more detail in the next chapter), so it's worth finding something that works for you now.

I'm struggling with pain in my pelvis

Given the amount of pressure that is sent down through the pelvis during pregnancy, the fact that your hormones are allowing your pelvis to be more mobile and how altered your walking/ sitting/sleeping are by your growing bump, it's hardly surprising that you might experience some pain or discomfort around the pelvic area. In fact, it is thought that around 50 per cent of women will experience some pelvic (or lower back) pain during pregnancy.[25]

However, pain in the pelvic area (including your lower back and upper legs) could well be a sign of pelvic girdle pain, which isn't always a straightforward 'it's-just-because-of-your-pregnancy-hormones' situation. Pelvic girdle pain is quite common during pregnancy and thought to affect around one in five women; you can read all about it on p. 213, and please do seek help as soon as possible from your health professional, as getting support early on can make a huge difference.

Regardless of the cause of pelvic pain, you do not have to stop moving your body. In fact, sitting down for too long and not being physically active may make it worse.

So it's all about assessing your triggers and finding alternatives or tweaks. For example, you may find that any movement or exercise that requires you to have your legs spread wide can make your pain worse. In that case, an exercise like skaters (where you jump from one end of your mat to the other, taking your legs wide) might not be one that works for you. Instead, you could switch to shorter side steps, or grapevine (yes, like the dance move!).

In essence, don't feel that pain requires bedrest. Definitely get checked over and definitely listen to your body; but also try to work out what aggravates or elevates your pain – and it may not be movement that does so.

I'm finding jumping/impact uncomfortable

During pregnancy, there is no known reason why you can't allow a little impact into your training, such as a jumping jack or squat jump. If you think about running, having sex, playing with your children, they will all involve a level of bouncing around and your baby is happily cushioned in your uterus so as to be ok with that. However, there may come a point where impact just doesn't feel right for you. Maybe you're finding that your chest is sore when you bounce around, or maybe your pelvic floor is struggling with the extra demand . . .

This is the time to tweak your exercises. There are low-impact versions (regressions) of all the Sweat exercises in The Bump Plan, so do make use of those. Sometimes you just have to park the ego and acknowledge that you'll be able to get back to impact exercises in the future – and probably that little bit sooner if you listen to your body now.

What is the focus in weeks 28–33?

Unless you have a contraindication (as discussed on p. 30), this is the time to really stick with it – staying physically active now might feel more challenging but will be so worth it. If you can continue through this phase, you'll be better equipped to stay active in the final push (weeks 34–40) and this can really help with preparing your body for labour. We'll discuss this concept (optimal foetal positioning) more in the next chapter, but there is a lot you can do to help your chances of a smoother labour (whether vaginal or Caesarean) by being active in this third trimester.

I like to use the third trimester to start looking ahead to what life will be like with a newborn and make sure I'm strong enough to deal with that. Think hours of cuddling, feeding and looking down at your lovely baby, pushing buggies and leaning over cots, all of which require some serious endurance and strength in the upper and mid-back – so we'll be making sure that arms and backs are ready for the job.

And don't forget that pelvic floor. By now it's got a huge job – it might be starting to get tired and you may be starting to notice it struggling. Do not give up on your pelvic floor exercises; they are so important, and any effort you put in now will help with your postnatal recovery, too (win–win).

Your exercises: weeks 28–33

Your warm-up and cool-down exercises can be found on pp. 74–76 and 87–88. Let's get started with your exercises for the first half of your third (and final) trimester.

Strength exercises

Single calf raises (suitable for TTC, entire pregnancy, if comfortable, and postnatal phases 1 and 2)

Single calf raises help to build strength in the calves (perhaps rather obviously), which can be really beneficial in reducing impact when you run, jog, bounce.

1. Stand with feet hip-width apart with arms extended to the side.
2. Come up into a calf raise with both feet and find your balance.
3. Shift your weight over to your right foot as much as you feel safe to do so.
4. Inhale to lower the right heel to the floor.
5. Exhale to lift the right heel back up into a calf raise.
6. Repeat on the other side.

TIP: As you rise up into the calf raise, try to keep the ankle as neutral as possible. It's going to want to buckle to the sides, potentially, but it's better to have good technique than to go as high as possible.

REGRESSION: try holding on to a chair or wall to help with your balance, or keep the weight more evenly spread across both legs.

PROGRESSION: you could try taking the other foot completely off the floor (so you are literally standing on one leg), but you may want to hold on to something for this version, as it's very wobbly!

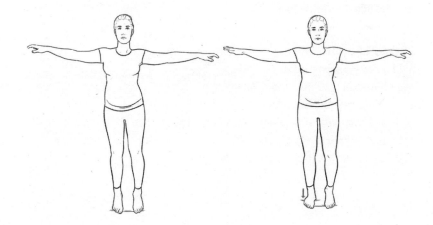

Rowing (suitable for TTC, entire pregnancy, if comfortable, and postnatal, all phases)

I honestly think that everyone should perform a version of rowing every day. It is such a great exercise for balancing out the shoulders and building strength in the upper back, which is particularly important ahead of your baby arriving.

1. In a seated, standing or kneeling position, start with the arms reaching out in front of you, at shoulder height, palms facing down and hands shoulder-width apart.
2. Inhale and, as you exhale, start to bend your arms, elbows pointing backwards, keeping them at shoulder height, and gently squeeze between the shoulder blades.
3. Inhale to take them back to the start position.
4. Repeat.

TIP: Try not to pop your ribcage forwards as you draw the arms back; this is about the shoulder blades moving around the sides and back of the ribcage and keeping the spine neutral and stable where possible.

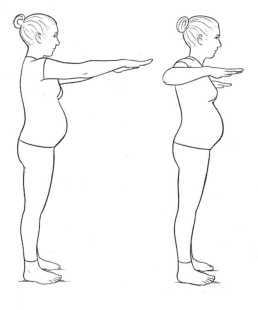

REGRESSION: simply slow the movement down and reduce the range to a manageable level.

PROGRESSION: you can hold a resistance band in your hands as you pull the arms back (try to keep your hands in line with your elbows as you do this, so the band is stretched); or hold a dumbbell in each hand. You can also try this movement in a half-hip hinge position to add extra demand to the postural chain.

Reverse flies (suitable for TTC, entire pregnancy, if comfortable, and postnatal, all phases)

Similar to rowing, reverse flies are great for preparing the shoulders and upper back for the demands of life with a newborn. There's going to be lots of holding and cuddling, so you'll need a strong back to manage that!

1. These can be performed seated, standing or kneeling, but in this version, I'd love you to try them in a half-hip hinge position.
2. Start with the arms extended out in front of you, palms facing each other, in line with the shoulders and elbows soft.
3. Inhale and, as you exhale, start to draw the arms back, without changing their shape, and gently squeeze between the shoulder blades.
4. Inhale to let the arms come back to their start position.

TIP: The similarity between this exercise and rowing is that you want some movement of the shoulder blades – they should gently squeeze towards each other; the difference is that in reverse flies the arms don't change shape – the elbows stay soft, but they do not bend.

REGRESSION: choose an easier start position (such as seated), rather than half-hip hinge, which is more challenging to the postural chain. Reduce the range of movement or slow the movement down.

PROGRESSION: hold on to a resistance band and pull on it as you open out the arms; or hold a dumbbell in each hand.

Superman (suitable for TTC, entire pregnancy, if comfortable, and postnatal phases 1 and 2)

Who doesn't love a superman (or superwoman) exercise? However, I do see these performed incorrectly an awful lot, which will recruit the wrong muscles, so do read my tips below.

1. Start on hands and knees, hands shoulder-width apart and knees hip-width apart, with a nice, neutral spine.
2. Maintaining your neutral spine, start to extend your left arm and right leg away from each other.
3. Inhale to release back to your start position.
4. Repeat with the right arm and left leg.

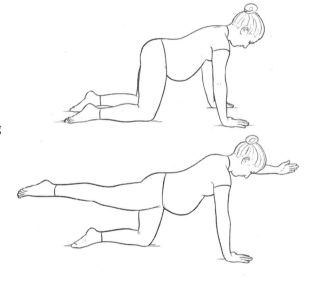

TIP: This is about maintaining a neutral, stable spine – not about how high you can get your hand and foot. If you notice your ribcage flaring or your lower back becoming uncomfortable you have gone too high and/or need to engage your core a little more. This exercise shouldn't look sexy – it should actually look quite boring and easy.

REGRESSION: choose to either move just the arm or just the leg at first, until you get used to the height you can take them to without losing your neutral spine.

PROGRESSION: hold a dumbbell in the hand you are reaching forwards; or, rather than doing one repetition before swapping sides, do a number of them with one arm and leg, then swap to the other arm and leg.

Pilates tricep push-ups (suitable for TTC, entire pregnancy, if comfortable, and postnatal phases 1 and 2)

These are a great way to build strength around the shoulder and in the upper back, but do adjust your start position to meet you where you are at right now.

1. These can be performed on hands and knees (four-point kneeling), half-plank (as illustrated) or full-plank (just ensure you are managing your pressure, whichever option you choose). Hands should be shoulder-width apart, elbows slightly soft with the elbow creases pointing forwards, and you need a nice, neutral spine.

2. As you inhale, start to bend your elbows, (keeping them tight to the sides of the ribcage as you do so), lowering your body down towards the floor while maintaining your neutral spine.

3. Exhale to press into the hands and slowly come back up to your start position.

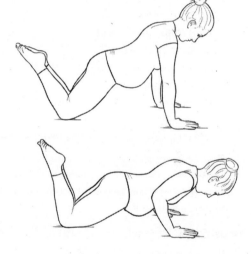

TIP: This is a tricep push-up, not a pec push-up, so keep the elbows pointing back towards your knees as they bend. Try to keep a nice, neutral spine as you move; if you can't, you'll need to regress the exercise to protect your back.

REGRESSION: the easiest option here is four-point kneeling, and you can then also shift some more weight out of the arms and into the legs to reduce the challenge. Try reducing the range of movement also; you do not have to get your nose to the floor – ok?

PROGRESSION: the hardest option here is to complete the exercise in a full-plank position, but you must be sure you are maintaining a neutral spine and are managing the pressure in your core (for more on this, see p. 174).

Sweat exercises

Squat kicks (suitable for TTC, entire pregnancy, if comfortable, and postnatal phase 2)

Feel free to choose between a parallel squat or a sumo squat here, depending on which is more comfortable for you at this stage of pregnancy.

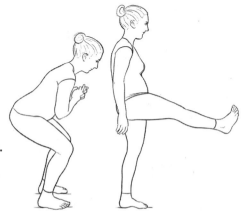

1. Stand, feet either hip-width apart and parallel or wider than hip-width and turned out (sumo squat), and hands in prayer position.
2. Squat down, stand up and kick your right leg out in front of you.
3. Squat down, stand up and kick your left leg out in front of you.

TIP: Aim for a nice, neutral spine as you move here, which will mean a slight hinge forwards as you squat down, and not too much leaning back at the top as you kick.

REGRESSION: feel free to get rid of the kick here, if you prefer; or simply lift the heel off the floor, rather than kicking the leg out.

PROGRESSION: hold a dumbbell in each hand; or try to lift your kicking leg off the floor before you get to the top of the squat to make it slightly more unstable (and hence more challenging).

Overhead reaches (suitable for TTC, entire pregnancy, if comfortable, and postnatal phase 2)

I love this exercise, as it promotes a little bit of spine extension (which most of us need more of), involves looking up (we spend so much time looking down) and it's low impact.

1. Stand, feet hip-width apart.
2. Reach your right arm up overhead, look up to where you are reaching and tap your right foot out to the side.
3. Bring the arm and foot back in, then reach the left arm up overhead and tap your left foot out to the side.

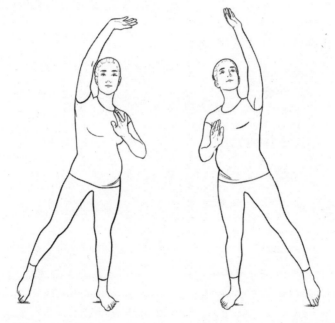

TIP: Really do stretch the arm up as high as you can to get the shoulder blade moving and think about the spine lengthening up towards the ceiling.

REGRESSION: simply slow the movement down.

PROGRESSION: pick up the pace; or hold a dumbbell in each hand.

Squat knee lifts (suitable for TTC, entire pregnancy, if comfortable, and postnatal phase 2)

Feel free to do this exercise in parallel, if you prefer, but it is easier to navigate a bump in a sumo squat position.

1. Stand, feet either hip-width apart and parallel or wider than hip-width and turned out (sumo squat), and hands in a fist position at your chest (as if ready to fight).
2. Squat down, stand up and lift your right knee up and outwards towards your right shoulder and rotate towards it.
3. Lower the leg and squat back down.
4. Stand up and lift your left knee up and outwards towards your left shoulder and rotate towards it.
5. Lower the leg back to start.

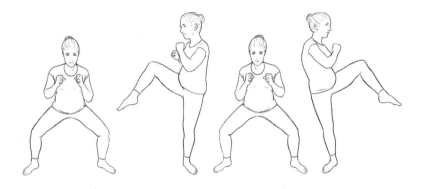

TIP: Try to maintain a nice, neutral spine as you do this exercise, and think about the shape you are creating with your body.

REGRESSION: feel free to remove the knee lift altogether, if you prefer – don't take the knee as high or simply lift the heel off the floor instead.

PROGRESSION: hold a dumbbell in each hand to add resistance, lift the knee higher or pick up the pace.

Curtsy lunges (suitable for TTC, entire pregnancy, if comfortable, and postnatal phase 2)

A great, dynamic exercise for the legs; and because your legs are in turnout here, you have a little more space for a growing bump to fit through.

1. Stand at the top of your mat, legs together in turnout (so heels together and toes out) and hands in prayer position.
2. Step your left foot back behind you, as if you are about to curtsy, and bend both knees to drop low to the floor.
3. Press through your right leg to push yourself up to standing.
4. Repeat on the other side.

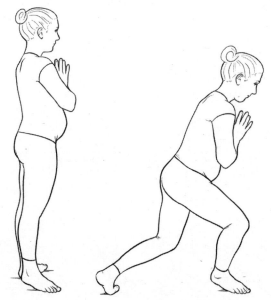

TIP: Aim to keep your spine neutral as you do this – this requires a slight hinge forwards as you curtsy. And press through your front leg to come back to standing, rather than pushing off the back leg.

REGRESSION: instead of stepping the leg back to curtsy, you could start in a lunge position and simply lower down and push up, rather than resetting each time.

PROGRESSION: hold a dumbbell in each hand to add resistance; or pick up the pace.

Squat jab rotations (suitable for TTC, entire pregnancy, if comfortable, and postnatal phase 2)

If you have any anger or frustration in your body right now, this exercise will feel great. If not (wow, lucky you!), ensure that these are proper energy-fuelled punches.

1. Start in your chosen squat start position (parallel feet, hip-width apart or sumo squat position, feet wider than hip-width and in turnout).
2. Squat down, stand up and rotate to the left while punching with your right hand.
3. Squat down, stand up and rotate to the right and punch with your left hand.

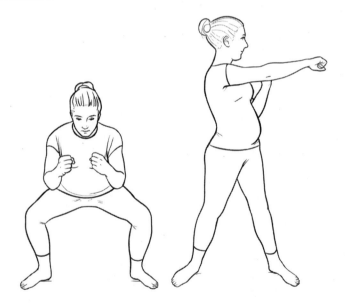

TIP: Aim for good squat technique here – sometimes we can be so distracted by the speed or choreography of a move that we forget our fundamentals. Imagine that you are going to sit down on a chair or toilet and maintain a nice, neutral spine.

REGRESSION: reduce the depth of the squat, reduce the speed or remove the punches, if need be.

PROGRESSION: add a dumbbell into each hand or pick up the pace.

Example routines

Below, you'll find two example routines. Routine 1 combines all of the exercise options. Routine 2 combines all of the Sweat exercises with a rest period (which you do not have to utilise). Feel free to repeat the routines to help you build up to the recommended 150 minutes of physical activity per week (an example week could be 5 x 30 minute workouts).

Routine 1

- *Warm-up*
- Squat kicks: 30–60 seconds
- Single calf raises: 30–60 seconds
- Overhead reaches: 30–60 seconds
- Rowing: 30–60 seconds
- Squat knee lifts: 30–60 seconds
- Reverse flies: 30–60 seconds
- Curtsy lunges: 30–60 seconds
- Superman: 30–60 seconds
- Squat jab rotations: 30–60 seconds
- Pilates tricep push-ups: 30–60 seconds
- *Repeat or cool-down* (if repeating, don't exceed four sets and be sure to include a rest period if you need it between sets)

Routine 2

- *Warm-up*
- Squat kicks: 30–60 seconds
- Rest – marching on the spot: 60 seconds
- Overhead reaches: 30–60 seconds
- Rest – marching on the spot: 60 seconds
- Squat knee lifts: 30–60 seconds

- Rest – marching on the spot: 60 seconds
- Curtsy lunges: 30–60 seconds
- Rest – marching on the spot: 60 seconds
- Squat jab rotations: 30–60 seconds
- *Repeat or cool-down* (if repeating, don't exceed four sets and be sure to include a rest period if you need it between sets)

Your pelvic floor exercise

The lift

This visualisation does what it says on the tin – you'll be imagining your pelvic floor as if it's a lift in a tall block of flats. The aim here is to help you get the most out of your pelvic floor lifts. It can also help to visualise the release phase of a pelvic floor contraction – imagining heading down to the basement of the tower block.

1. Start in a comfortable position – this might be seated, lying, side-lying, standing.
2. Close your eyes (this will help you to focus internally) and try to clear your mind.
3. Focus on your breathing by bringing your awareness to breathing in and out through your nose. Relax your jaw and ensure your tongue is relaxed in your mouth.
4. Imagine that your pelvic floor is currently on the ground floor of a tower block, ensuring it is relaxed to start. Inhale and imagine the pelvic floor going down a floor, into the basement and, as you exhale, imagine the pelvic floor going up to the very top of the tower by lifting and contracting it.
5. Then, as you inhale, imagine your pelvic floor coming back down to the basement of the tower block by releasing it fully.
6. Exhale to lift back to the top floor again.
7. Repeat 8–10 times.

TIP: When releasing the pelvic floor to the 'basement', you're not trying to bear down on it (as you would to pass urine), but simply encouraging a release of the contraction you have just created. Don't panic if you can't *feel* this release; as always, it's more about the concept or awareness of releasing the pelvic floor after contracting it.

What is pelvic girdle pain?

by Dr Sinéad Dufour, professor and pelvic health physiotherapist

If you've started to experience pain in the lower back and pubic area when you change position, sit or stand for longer periods, you might – understandably – be concerned. The pain might make it very difficult for you to function; perhaps you're worried about whether you can continue to work or fearful about the upcoming birth of your baby and whether you will be able to care for them.

This pain presentation is referred to as pregnancy-related pelvic girdle pain (PPGP) and is an umbrella term covering pain in the symphysis pubis joint (the front of the pelvis) and the sacroiliac joints (at the back of the pelvis). PPGP is usually characterised by tension and guarding around the pelvis, including the pelvic floor. Minor aches and pains through the lower back and pelvis are to be expected in pregnancy, but PPGP – although common – can be debilitating. The tissues and structures around the pelvis will feel sensitive and sore. It is not because structures are unstable or that there is 'dysfunction' of any pelvic structures, but your previous experiences, current health status, and state of mind play a role. For many, the pain does ease off when baby is born but, for others, it can continue in the postpartum period.

The following risk factors might make you more suscepti-ble to PPGP:

- Parity – meaning having had a baby previously (PPGP does not often happen in a first pregnancy).
- Previous trauma of any form (a very high proportion of women experience trauma birthing their first baby).
- Previous history of lower back or pelvic pain (a situa-tion which will alter sensory distribution and make PPGP more likely).
- Increased body-mass index (BMI) – this can cause systemic inflammation which contributes to the pelvis becoming more sensitive.
- Smoking – again, this causes inflammation.
- Lack of belief in improvement – this one is huge, as one's understanding of their symptoms will dictate the course of their recovery (many women are led to believe that PPGP is related to the pregnancy itself when it isn't; it is related to the context of the person beyond their pregnancy).

The points listed above show that PPGP can largely be brought on by psychological factors, and is not necessarily caused by the biology of pregnancy, per se. If you had a diffi-cult first birth or a challenging time in the postpartum period and you have lingering fears related to birth, it is understandable that your pain-alarm system will start going off in a subsequent pregnancy.

Tackling fear related to aspects of pregnancy, birth and postpartum and fear related to movement, therefore, is key.

A common misunderstanding is that pain with movement means the movement is 'damaging', which is far from true. One oft-suggested PPGP treatment is to brace and tighten your legs and tummy to 'hold everything together' but this will, in fact, only make things worse. As you know from reading this book so far, it's beneficial for mamas to move! Thankfully, there are lots of ways to adapt movement and to train the nervous system to be in a less threatened state. If you think you're experiencing PPGP, look for a pelvic health physiotherapist who'll help you to manage any negative feelings you're holding on to from previous experiences, as well as work with you to find ways of moving that are comfortable. With the right guidance, PPGP can be resolved and self-managed.

Pregnancy weeks 34–40+

We're at the final push now (pun entirely intended!).

This section will take you all the way through to your labour, and I am so happy you're still here with me.

I'm writing this at 38 weeks pregnant myself, so I know how some of you might be feeling (although of course we're all different). I'm feeling pretty squashed, I'm weeing about 5 times an hour, I've actually fractured a rib coughing this week (to be fair, it was a bad chest infection) and sleep is not my friend. However, I am beyond excited that at any time I might feel a sign that my baby is on their way, and I hope you're feeling positive, too.

In this last phase, I want to really manage expectations. The physical activity guidelines are still the same as they were in week 1 of pregnancy, but you'll be a different person right now. You'll have a very heavy bump, you might be struggling to breathe deeply and you might find your pelvic floor is a little more challenged than you'd like – so don't beat yourself up if you have to slow things down a little. As always, listen to your body and do the activity and exercises you enjoy. Staying active in this final phase can really help to get your body ready for labour and your baby into a great position for birth; and it can also help you to manage your mental health. So let's give it a go!

Your body

In week 34, your baby weighs around 2.5kg (which, if it was a dumbbell in your hand, for example, would get pretty tiring, pretty quickly). It's a substantial weight, and that's just the baby itself – that doesn't include their extensive entourage of amniotic fluid, placenta and more. It's also around 45cm long (about the size of a backpack), so it's taking up a huge amount of space in your abdominal cavity. For this reason, you might find your pelvic floor is feeling the pressure, your linea alba is stretched and you have some level of diastasis recti going on (remember this is a functional part of pregnancy) and find it harder to breathe deeply. Essentially, your baby is taking up a lot of space and there are bound to be repercussions.

Here are some of the main symptoms at this stage:

- **A reduction in symptoms.** Yes, you read that right. At some point in the coming weeks, you may find some of your symptoms reduce slightly. This can be caused by your baby starting to drop down into the pelvis and engaging, allowing you a sense of having more room again.
- **Rib pain.** We've talked about this one before but, understandably, it is common at this stage of pregnancy, as your uterus is so high up in the ribcage. If your baby is head down (which 95 per cent of babies are by the time of delivery), you may feel some kicks to the old ribs every now and again, too.

- **Nesting.** Not a physical symptom as such, but a common occurrence near the end of pregnancy. The desire to tidy, clean, organise, wash clothes is strong for so many at this stage. And remember that housework counts towards your physical activity minutes, too – so it's a win–win!
- **Boredom or frustration.** Again, more of a mental health symptom, rather than a physical one. If you've gone over your due date or you're simply impatient to meet your little one, you may find that frustration really sinks in. Try and stay busy if you can – meet friends, book a massage (if funds allow), or go to the cinema (it's so much harder to do these things once you're a parent).
- **Insomnia.** It feels so cruel, and when people tell you, 'It's your body preparing you for when the baby arrives', you want to bite their heads off, but sadly, insomnia can rear its ugly head at this stage. Get a good book or start a new TV series and try to go with the flow, if you can.

What you need to know

The way you move your body during pregnancy is thought to influence the positioning of your baby, and thus your labour. I find this fascinating. Also, knowing that you might be able to do something in these last few weeks to benefit your labour experience can be really motivating and positive, at a time where some can feel a little helpless. At best, you may improve your birth experience, and at worst it will make no difference – so I think it's worth giving it a go.

In this final phase, your baby will be doing some wriggling and jiggling to (hopefully) get themselves into the right position for birth. Now some of you will be planning a vaginal birth, while others may be planning a Caesarean. I will be talking a fair amount about vaginal birth in the next few paragraphs, but please know that there is no judgment here (Freya and Kit were both born by Caesarean).

In the coming weeks, most babies will work their way down into the pelvis (which we call engaging), ready for birth. As mentioned, it's thought that there are a few things you can do to allow this process to run smoothly and help your baby to get into the best possible position. It can help to understand the mechanics of the pelvis first, though.

When we rotate our legs outwards in the hip sockets, turning our knees and toes away from each other, we call this external rotation. Now external rotation causes the top of the pelvis (the pelvic inlet) to get wider and slightly expand. This could be helpful in allowing the baby to make its way down into the pelvis and engage. Chances are your baby will only do this when they are good and ready (they're stubborn little things), but squats in external rotation, for example, could help.

When we rotate our legs inwards in the hip sockets, turning our knees and toes towards each other, we call this medial rotation. This movement causes the base of the pelvis to grow wider and expand, essentially pulling the sit bones apart. This can be helpful during delivery and so labour positions that encourage medial rotation (or knees in and feet out) could help support a vaginal birth.

What about optimal foetal positioning?

Optimal foetal positioning is the theory that getting your baby into the best possible position for either a vaginal or Caesarean birth could improve labour. That position is called occiput-anterior (OA), and it's where the baby's head is down (and their feet are up), and they are facing your spine (so they are the reverse of you). In this position, the baby is thought to have the most straightforward passage through the pelvis during a vaginal birth, potentially reducing the chances of an emergency Caesarean (although please remember you can do everything 'by the book' and things can still change during labour). This all sounds fantastic, right? And I'm sure we are all on board with anything that could make things smoother on the day. Sign me up . . .

How can I encourage optimal foetal positioning?
It's possible that spending time in certain poses may improve the chances of your baby being in this position. The heaviest part of a baby is its back, and it will naturally deviate towards gravity. Therefore, any position that encourages their back to move towards your front could be beneficial. Let's take, for example, hands-and-knees position: here, gravity could help draw the baby's back down towards the floor, which would help them to be facing your spine (OA – see above). This would be the same for any 'prone' position (where you are facing the floor or leaning forwards).

What is the focus in weeks 34–40+?

Anything you manage to do at this stage (from a physical activity point of view) is fantastic. Keeping your body moving, getting out into fresh air and not spending too much time being sedentary are all important, if you can manage.

You'll notice that your pelvic floor exercise in this phase is all about pelvic floor relaxation. This is because it needs to be both strong and flexible to be functional, and this means it has to be able to contract and stretch. If you are hoping for a vaginal birth, there will come a point in labour when your pelvic floor muscles stretch and lengthen as the baby passes through, with some of them stretching up to 3.26 times their original length.[26] It can be beneficial, therefore, for your pelvic floor to be capable of relaxing and allowing the stretch to happen, rather than being tight and tense.

So in your pelvic floor exercise, you'll be visualising that lengthening occurring, using your breath and your mind–body connection. That last part might sound a bit woo-woo, but really, it's just consciously being aware of what is going on in the body; essentially, it means concentrating, and not just muscling through an exercise mindlessly. You may not *feel* anything, but it's the awareness of what you are trying to achieve that matters.

You'll notice that some of the Strength exercises in this section involve medial rotation of the leg (reverse clams and squats with medial rotation). Thinking back to what you've read above, practising this type of movement could be helpful for any upcoming vaginal births. Remember, medial rotation is a great labour position, so whether standing, kneeling or side-lying, it's a good idea to get used to it.

Your exercises: weeks 34–40+

Your warm-up and cool-down exercises can be found on pp. 74–76 and 87–88. You're nearly there! Now let's get into your final set of Strength and Sweat pregnancy exercises.

Strength exercises

Squats with medial rotation (suitable for TTC, entire pregnancy, if comfortable, and postnatal phases 1 and 2)

This is a great way to get in some medial rotation of the leg, especially if you know you spend a lot of time with your feet pointing outwards!

1. Stand with your feet parallel and hip-width apart (or slightly wider) and hands in prayer position.
2. Squat down, maintaining a nice, neutral spine, and keeping your knees pointing forwards.
3. As you exhale, bring your knees towards each other, rotating the legs inwards.
4. As you inhale, bring the knees back to parallel.
5. Repeat.

TIP: This is all about endurance, as you stay in the squat for the duration of the exercise. Warning: you will feel the burn! Make sure that the leg is rotating in the hip socket, and you aren't just squeezing your thighs together.

REGRESSION: you can do one repetition (legs rotate inwards) and then stand up each time, so that you aren't held in a squat position for as long. You can also practise this in a much higher squat position or standing (although it's a bit awkward).

PROGRESSION: hold a dumbbell in each hand to add resistance (it makes you heavier); or add a 10-second hold at the end (legs turned inwards) or a 10-second pulse (legs turned inwards and little bounces).

Hip hikes (suitable for TTC, entire pregnancy, if comfortable, and postnatal phases 1 and 2)

Hip hikes are great for those who tend to drop their hips to one side or the other or struggle to maintain a level pelvis when one leg is lifted off the floor. They challenge the hip abductors in a really functional way.

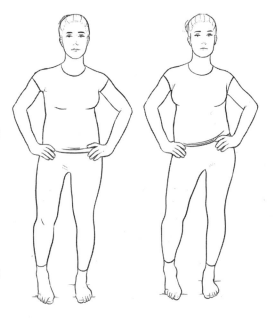

1. Stand with the feet hip-width apart and hands on your hips.
2. Shift your weight over to the left leg and lift your right heel off the floor.
3. Keeping your left leg straight (but not locked), try to drop your right hip downwards, so your pelvis is no longer level.
4. Press into your left leg to bring the right hip back up.
5. Repeat as required and then swap legs.

TIP: You are trying to drop your hip here and then correct it – so really visualise the pelvis tilting from side to side. If you are struggling with pelvic girdle pain (see p. 213) and this exercise is triggering, I'd advise avoiding it.

REGRESSION: keep the weight more equally spread across both feet, rather than loading the standing leg so much.

PROGRESSION: try lifting your foot off the floor completely (rather than just the heel), so that you lose your base of support and the pelvis is even heavier to lift.

Reverse clams (suitable for TTC, entire pregnancy, if comfortable, and postnatal phases 1 and 2)

I absolutely love reverse clams, especially at this stage of pregnancy, as they can really help to boost pelvic stability.

1. Lie on your left-hand side, left arm extended along the floor to be used as a pillow, knees bent to around 90˚, heels in line with your tailbone and hips stacked.
2. Inhale and, as you exhale, lift your right foot up towards the ceiling, keeping your knees together, taking your leg into medial rotation (turned inwards).
3. Inhale to lower the foot back down.
4. Repeat as required, and then swap legs.

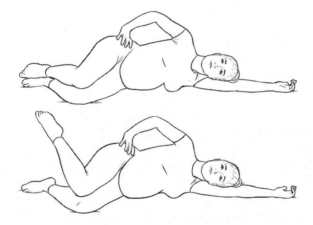

TIP: This exercise is about the leg rotating within the hip socket, not the pelvis itself rotating, so try to keep the spine and pelvis nice and still. Visualise the leg turning within the ball-and-socket hip joint.

REGRESSION: simply slow the movement down or reduce the range of movement.

PROGRESSION: tie a resistance band or loop around your ankles; you can also try to hover your top knee a few centimetres or so away from your bottom knee and perform the same movement, to challenge your endurance.

Cat-cows (suitable for TTC, entire pregnancy, if comfortable, and postnatal phases 1 and 2)

Cat-cows usually feel fantastic, as they get the spine moving. If you use this postnatally, just be mindful of how it feels on any new scars – it should feel comfortable.

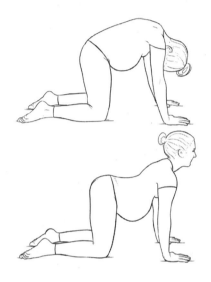

1. Start on hands and knees, with hands shoulder-width apart, knees hip-width apart and a nice, neutral spine.
2. Inhale and, as you exhale, start to flex and round your spine into an angry cat position, bringing your nose towards your knees.
3. As you inhale, come back past neutral and take your spine into extension, lifting your tailbone and the crown of your head up towards the ceiling to achieve a cow-like position.
4. Repeat.

TIP: Ideally, you want the entire spine to move here, but what most people will find is that one part will move a lot, while another will stay quite rigid. I recommend sending your focus and intention to that rigid area, so that hopefully, over time, it opens up slightly, too.

REGRESSION: if you find this is uncomfortable for your wrists, you can sit your weight back into your legs a little more and make the hands lighter on the floor.

PROGRESSION: there isn't really a progression here other than really focusing on the shapes you are creating, maybe using a mirror or videoing your technique to review.

Cactus (suitable for TTC, entire pregnancy, if comfortable, and postnatal, all phases)

Cactus is up there as one of my go-to exercises for all my clients, as it helps to balance out the shoulders and build strength in the upper back – a winner ahead of your newborn arriving.

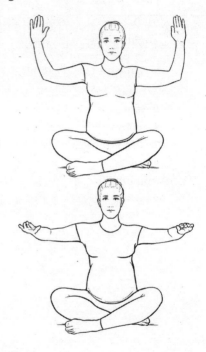

1. This can be performed standing, seated or kneeling, starting with a neutral spine, arms lifted out to crucifix, palms facing forwards and shoulders relaxed.
2. Lift and bend your arms, so that your shoulders and elbows are both at around 90° and you look a little like a cactus.
3. Inhale and rotate the arms in the shoulder sockets until the palms face the floor and the forearms are parallel to the floor/horizontal.
4. Exhale and rotate the arms back to their start position, aiming to bring the forearms back to vertical.
5. Repeat.

TIP: This exercise is all about rotation of the arm in the shoulder, so try to avoid moving the rest of the body as the arms move. Focus on the backward rotation of the arms, as this is the juicy bit – it is what most of us need more of in our lives.

REGRESSION: you may find that your upper traps take over, so feel free to rest and have a quick wriggle before jumping back into it if needed. You could also try having your elbows a little lower.

PROGRESSION: hold a dumbbell in each hand to add extra resistance.

Sweat exercises

Fast punches (suitable for TTC, entire pregnancy, if comfortable, and postnatal phase 2)

Another great exercise for those days when you have some aggression to release or some energy to burn.

1. Start in your chosen squat start position (feet parallel and hip-width apart or sumo squat), hands in fists by your chest, as if ready to fight.
2. Start punching with the arms alternating for each punch, keeping your bottom as still as possible.

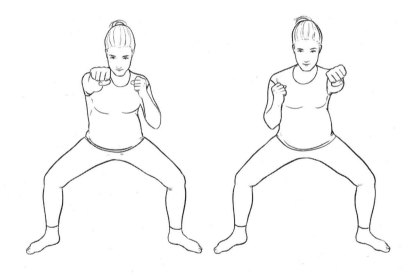

TIP: This is a great endurance exercise for the lower half, but also challenges your stability, if you can keep everything else nice and still.

REGRESSION: you could remove the squat and do this standing; or take regular rests standing, if needed, before dropping back down into a squat.

PROGRESSION: add a dumbbell in each hand for extra resistance.

Modified split punches (suitable for TTC, entire pregnancy, if comfortable, and postnatal phases 1 and 2)

This is a low-impact version of the split punches on p. 183. You may still feel happy bouncing around at this stage of your pregnancy, but I personally prefer this version at this point.

1. Stand with feet hip-width apart and hands at your chest in fists, as if ready for a fight.
2. Take your left foot and tap it out in front of you, while taking your right arm and punching it forwards.
3. Bring the leg and arm back in and switch to repeat with the right foot and left arm.

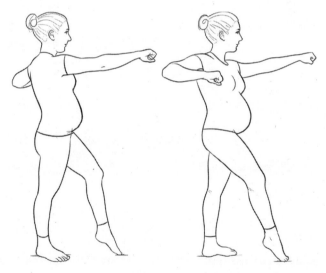

TIP: Try to stand nice and neutral as you do this, rather than hunching over as you punch, or leaning back as you switch legs. Make sure the punches are 'proper' ones with energy behind them.

REGRESSION: you could either do the leg element of this exercise or the arm element, rather than both together.

PROGRESSION: hold a dumbbell in each hand for extra resistance; or use the higher-impact version of this exercise on p. 183.

Diamonds (suitable for TTC, entire pregnancy, if comfortable, and postnatal phase 2)

This is a great exercise for strengthening the postural chain (the muscles that run up the back of the body and keep you upright). If you find that your bump is in the way, simply reduce the range of movement – you don't have to touch your ankle here.

1. Stand with feet parallel and as wide as is comfortable for your pelvis, arms extended to the side at shoulder height and a nice, neutral spine.
2. Bend your left knee, hinge forward at your hips, rotate your upper body towards your left leg and reach your right arm across towards your left foot.
3. Straighten your left leg to bring yourself back to your start position.
4. Repeat on the other side.

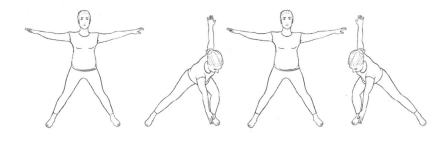

TIP: Aim to keep your spine quite neutral here, so it is almost like a hip hinge, rather than hunching over to get lower. Bring the arms back to shoulder height each time, so that the deltoids (those triangular shoulder muscles) get a good workout, too.

REGRESSION: simply perform the leg element of the exercise, taking it into a side lunge, essentially. Arms can stay out to the sides, and you can keep your spine upright.

PROGRESSION: add a dumbbell in each hand for extra resistance.

Line taps (suitable for TTC, entire pregnancy, if comfortable, and postnatal phase 2)

This exercise reminds me of those freezing cold afternoons at school spent practising hockey or netball drills, running from one painted line to another. There was a reason we were made to do them, though, sadly, so I'm passing these on to you.

1. Stand at the right end of your mat in a squat position, reaching your left hand down, as if touching a line on the floor.
2. Staying low, quickly side-step your way to the other end of your mat and pretend to reach for the floor with your right hand.

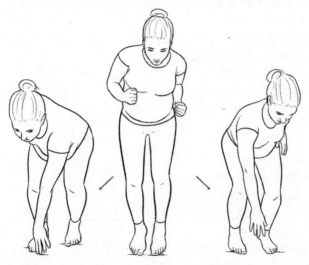

TIP: If your bump is in the way here, don't worry. You don't actually have to touch the floor – just drop as low as is comfortable for you, maintaining a neutral spine (try not to hunch over just to get lower).

REGRESSION: come up to standing to shimmy to the other end of the mat each time, rather than staying low.

PROGRESSION: you could tie a resistance band around your ankles to add resistance for the shimmy element, but do slow the movement down slightly to prevent falling. You could also add a dumbbell in each hand – again, for extra resistance.

Modified floor to ceilings (suitable for TTC, entire pregnancy, if comfortable, and postnatal phase 2)

This is the low-impact version of the floor-to-ceiling exercise on p. 86. If you feel comfortable still jumping around, feel free to continue with that one, but I prefer the modified version at this stage of pregnancy.

1. Start in your chosen squat start position (either feet parallel and hip-width apart or sumo squat) and arms by your sides.
2. Squat down and imagine you are about to pick something up off the floor.
3. Stand up and reach your arms overhead, as if putting that same item up on a high shelf.
4. Repeat.

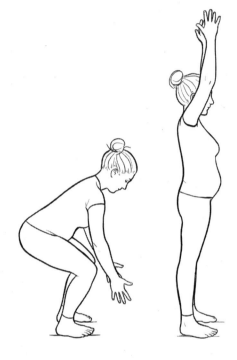

TIP: This is a great way to learn good lifting technique ahead of your little one's arrival and get into the habit of using your legs to lift you back up. Keep a neutral spine here throughout and make sure it is the legs bending that's bringing you closer to the floor (not your back rounding and hunching).

REGRESSION: reduce the range of movement or slow the pace right down.

PROGRESSION: you could add in a calf raise at the top, as you reach the arms overhead, or a jump, if that feels comfortable. You could also choose an item to actually pick up off the floor, as long as it isn't too heavy to maintain good form. Hold it with both hands – almost as if you are picking a box up off the floor.

Example routines

Below, you'll find two example routines. Routine 1 combines all of the exercise options. Routine 2 combines all of the Sweat exercises with a rest period (which you do not have to utilise). Feel free to repeat the routines to help you build up to the recommended 150 minutes of physical activity per week (an example week could be 5 x 30 minute workouts).

Routine 1

- *Warm-up*
- Fast punches: 30–60 seconds
- Squats with medial rotation: 30–60 seconds
- Modified split punches: 30–60 seconds
- Hip hikes: 30–60 seconds
- Diamonds: 30–60 seconds
- Reverse clams: 30–60 seconds
- Line taps: 30–60 seconds
- Cat-cows: 30–60 seconds
- Modified floor to ceilings: 30–60 seconds
- Cactus: 30–60 seconds
- *Repeat or cool-down* (if repeating, don't exceed four sets and be sure to include a rest period if you need it between sets)

Routine 2

- *Warm-up*
- Fast punches: 30–60 seconds
- Rest – marching on the spot: 60 seconds
- Modified split punches: 30–60 seconds
- Rest – marching on the spot: 60 seconds
- Diamonds: 30–60 seconds

- Rest – marching on the spot: 60 seconds
- Line taps: 30–60 seconds
- Rest – marching on the spot: 60 seconds
- Modified floor to ceilings: 30–60 seconds
- *Repeat or cool-down* (if repeating, don't exceed four sets and be sure to include a rest period if you need it between sets)

Your pelvic floor exercise

Pelvic floor relaxation

We've spent a lot of time working on contracting and strengthening the pelvic floor, and now is a good time to focus on how to relax it, as you approach your labour day. While this is more beneficial for those who end up having a vaginal birth (as the pelvic floor will need to relax during labour), it's a skill that will benefit everyone.

1. Start in a comfortable, *relaxing* position. This might be seated, lying or side-lying; or, if you are able to take your knees wide enough comfortably, child's pose is a really great position for this.
2. Close your eyes (this will help you to focus internally) and try to clear your mind.
3. Focus on your breathing by bringing your awareness to breathing in and out through your nose. Relax your jaw and ensure your tongue is relaxed in your mouth.
4. On your inhale, imagine the breath you take in is travelling down to your pelvic floor. (When you inhale, remember that the pelvic floor lengthens and relaxes, so visualise this if you can.)
5. On your exhale, simply breathe out – don't lift or squeeze, just exhale. (Remember that when you exhale, your pelvic floor will return to its start position.)
6. Repeat for 60–120 seconds.

TIP: This can be a tough exercise to get your head around, as you're not really *doing* anything. You're not actively lifting or squeezing or bearing down – you're just allowing the breath to do the work. Visualising the breath heading down to the pelvic floor can seem a bit woo-woo, but it might just stop some of you gripping through your pelvic floor when it should be relaxing.

Preparing for birth

by Emma Brockwell, pelvic health physiotherapist and author of
Why Did No One Tell Me?, *and Hollie Grant*

Emma Brockwell on preparing for a vaginal birth

One of the best ways you can prepare for a vaginal birth is by
practising perineal massage. You may have heard of it, but
maybe you haven't. Chances are someone is going to mention
it to you at some point, whether that's a friend, relative or
your midwife. But is perineal massage worth it? I'm going to
jump straight to the answer and say yes! However, surveys
have shown that many women do not know what perineal
massage is, or, if they do, they are often too embarrassed to
do it; and many do not know the benefits and therefore do
not consider it part of their antenatal self-care. There is also
uncertainty around how to do it. So let me take this opportunity to help you see that perineal massage is worth it – because,
quite simply, *you* are worth it.

What is perineal massage?

Perineal massage is the act of stretching the perineal tissues,
preparing them for childbirth and making them more 'elastic'.
This can be carried out from around 34 weeks pregnant for
around 3–4 minutes, 3–4 times a week.

Are there any benefits?

Absolutely! Let's be honest, one of the fears surrounding a
vaginal delivery is tearing. Ninety per cent of women will
experience some form of tearing around the perineum

during a vaginal delivery. This, of course, ranges from small grazes to more significant tears that require stitches. Perineal digital massage has been shown in studies[27] to reduce the likelihood of either tearing or having an episiotomy by around 9 per cent and also to reduce ongoing perineal pain (in women who have birthed vaginally before).

Even if you are planning on having a Caesarean section, I would still recommend perineal massage, just in case your baby decides to come a little earlier than planned and is delivered vaginally.

How do I do perineal massage?

- Start with a warm bath to help relax the area.
- Make sure your hands are clean before starting and that your nails are short.
- A great place to do this is on your bed. Sit upright and supported, bend your knees up and then let them fall out to the sides (you can support them with pillows).
- Massage a vaginal lubricant or almond (or olive) oil into your perineum.
- Gently place both thumbs (if both are too much, try just one) into the opening of your vagina (see diagram below) and rest your fingertips on your bottom.
- With a light pressure, press down towards the anus, until you feel a stretch (or light burning sensation). Hold for up to a minute.
- Now make a sweeping motion side to side. Visualise your vaginal canal as a clock with twelve o'clock being at your pubic bone and six at your rectum. You are stretching from three to nine, like a U.

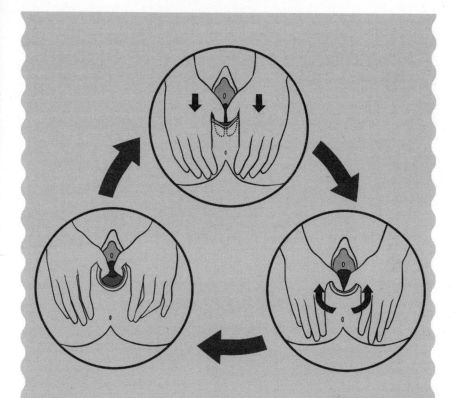

- The stretch will be intense but should not be painful. It should get easier as you practise.
- Keep relaxed and take deep breaths as you do this. And if you really do not want to do it yourself, you can ask your partner to help.

When not to do perineal massage

If you have had vaginal bleeding, an active infection or a ruptured membrane, do not carry out perineal massage without consulting your midwife or GP first.

If you are still unsure, you could even ask a pelvic health physiotherapist to guide you because this technique is so worth getting comfortable with. Yes, initially it does feel weird, but the benefits are very much worth it.

Hollie Grant on preparing for an elective Caesarean section
Spoiler alert: I (Hollie) have, at the time of writing this, now had two Caesarean sections – one emergency and one elective. The difference between the two couldn't be more stark, and I feel I've learned a lot along the way when it comes to dealing with previous birth trauma, preparing mentally and physically for surgery, planning and preparing for my recovery and navigating parenting post-Caesarean (parenting both a newborn and a toddler is no joke).

I feel strongly that all births should be incredibly beautiful events, and that a Caesarean birth can be a positive experience. So here are some of my thoughts for those planning an elective Caesarean – a brain dump of advice you might say! I hope it helps.

- Try to address any previous birth trauma ahead of time: if you are having an elective Caesarean after a previously traumatic birth (whether Caesarean or vaginal), I would really recommend you seek support for this as soon as you feel able. This might be in the form of a private birth-reflection session, requesting and reviewing your previous birth notes, therapy or simply opening up to friends or family. Doing the work ahead of your upcoming birth could make a huge difference to how you feel on the day, and your overall birth experience. You can read more about birth trauma on p. 268.

- Communicate with your midwife: the beauty of an elective Caesarean is that you have some notice (even if only short). This allows you time to communicate any concerns, wishes and questions to your midwife. For me, this meant I could explain what I found challenging with my first Caesarean and work out ways to mitigate this the second time around.

- Pack like a boss. Some of the items I used most from my hospital bag were: disposable maternity shorts/ adult incontinence pants (this meant that I could add maternity pads to them if needed, while also having something high waisted, clean and supportive to cover my scar), big maternity pads (yes, you still have post-natal bleeding, called Locchia, when you have a Caesarean), comfy loose trousers (so your scar isn't compressed) and chewing gum (trapped wind is common after a Caesarean and chewing gum can help).

- Prepare any siblings: I made sure I explained to Freya that I would be a little bit sore when I got home, that we could have lots of kisses but that cuddling might be a little tricky at first, that Daddy would be doing bath and bedtimes for a while (but not forever) and that she wouldn't be able to climb on me or be picked up by me for a while. I was lucky that she was old enough to understand, which really helped, and I think it was important she knew that how I felt initially wouldn't last forever!

- Experiment with your bed set-up: you know those popular bedside cots that strap to your side of the bed?

They're great – unless, that is, you have had a Caesarean and need to get out of bed to go to the toilet and have to shimmy down the bed to get past the cot! It's worth playing around with your bed/sleeping set-up before surgery, keeping in mind that you will be in some pain and that your mobility will be limited in the first few weeks.

- Read up on the surgery: not everyone will want to do this, but it can really help to find out what happens in a Caesarean, so you can be fully prepared for the sheer number of people in the room, what their jobs are, what the process is and what to expect.

Overall, I want you to know that the births of both my children were the happiest days of my life, and I would happily have a Caesarean every day for the rest of my life if I had to. I hope your Caesarean feels calm and positive, and that you have the support around you – both in surgery and postnatally – that you deserve.

And there you have it . . .

I hope you've found moving your body throughout your pregnancy a positive, empowering experience and that you're now approaching your baby's birth feeling like an absolute badass. You are stronger than you realise and can cope with anything that labour and parenting might throw your way. I know the next few days, or weeks, will be full of emotions, and I can't tell you how much I am thinking of all of you and your upcoming journey.

I hope you have the smoothest of journeys from here onwards, and I cannot wait to help you get back to the things you love most, postnatally. See you on the other side!

Part 3: Your Postnatal Workouts

Birth and your body

You've had a baby! Woah. There really are no words that can summarise how mind-bendingly, overwhelmingly surreal it is to become a parent. The immense cacophony of emotions, the shock and awe of what your body has just been through, and the terrifying pressure of looking after someone so small and helpless. Early motherhood can be intensely incredible and intensely challenging in equal measure. I hope that whatever you are experiencing, or feeling, you have support around you and feel comfortable accepting help when it's offered.

I say this not to be negative, or to scare anyone, but because I know from experience that the first weeks or months, even, can feel like a total daze, especially if there were any complications during labour or early on. It makes total sense that you might feel emotions other than purely positive ones, and I think we need to normalise the fact that motherhood can be tough. It doesn't mean you don't love your child or that you're a bad parent – it just means that it is hard.

Now I'm fairly sure you're reading this part of the book because you want to know how on earth you can piece your body back together again post labour. I speak to so many women who just don't know where to begin or what the guidelines are, and I admit that even I felt slightly nervous about 'doing the wrong thing' in those early days. I think I was slightly shocked by just how fragile I felt, and it hit home how monumental an event giving birth is, no matter how you do it.

The problem new parents face is that the guidance on postnatal exercise has traditionally been slightly limited and/or contradictory. There's also a myth that seems to linger that you shouldn't do any physical activity until you've had your 6-week check-up with your doctor, after which you can just crack on as you did pre-conception. Now anyone who has attended one of these appointments will know that it's short, a lot of the checks carried out are not on you but on your baby, and that your body/ stitches/diastasis or fitness goals are not always discussed or observed. Basically, do not expect that you'll have lots of time at that appointment to discuss how you'll get back to running a 10k – and even if you do, GPs are not always the most qualified to advise on postnatal fitness rehab (they can't be amazing at everything).

In fact, there's a lot you can do before the 6-week check-up to speed up and smooth out your postnatal recovery, and my aim here is to give you the facts about what is achievable, and help you rehabilitate your body and get back to the things you love doing, safely.

First, let's dive in and get an idea of what happened to you (no matter how long ago you gave birth), and where to begin with your postnatal recovery.

Vaginal birth – what happens to your body?

As someone who ended up with an emergency Caesarean with Freya, and an elective Caesarean with Kit, my initial reaction is to say "Congratulations" and "I'm so jealous" to anyone who has had a vaginal birth. But I know very well that a vaginal delivery can be incredible and simple for some, but traumatic and difficult for others. It's not black and white as to which type of birth is easiest to recover from, or least traumatising for the mother, so I hope that yours was as smooth as possible, a positive experience and that you're feeling supported by those around you.

However your vaginal birth went, there's one thing you all have in common – you pushed a baby out of your vagina. You are absolute warriors! But even the smoothest birth can have some side effects, so let's discuss some of the things that may have happened and require some consideration in your postnatal recovery.

Assisted vaginal delivery

Some of you may have experienced an assisted vaginal delivery, where a medical professional uses specially designed instruments – forceps and/or a ventouse – to help you give birth. Use of these instruments generally requires an episiotomy (see below) to create more space in the vaginal opening, and also increases your risk of tearing. It usually causes more postnatal bleeding in the immediate period following birth, but that should revert to the same as an unassisted vaginal birth very soon. In the UK, around one in eight women has an assisted vaginal birth, and this is more likely in those having their first baby (it goes up to one in three[1]).

The risk of a third- or fourth-degree tear (which we'll discuss in a moment) is increased during an assisted vaginal birth, as is urinary and/or anal incontinence (because of more severe tearing).

Tears and episiotomies

Up to 90 per cent of women will experience some form of tearing, grazing or episiotomy during a vaginal birth and these can vary in intensity and location.[2] Most of them will be around the perineum, which is the space between the vaginal opening and the anus, and most will be minor and heal quickly.

Tears

Types of tears can be broken down as follows:

- **First-degree tears.** These are small tears that only affect the skin. They usually heal naturally and don't require stitches. While they can be very sore, they shouldn't cause any long-term problems.
- **Second-degree tears.** These affect both the skin and muscle of the perineum. They usually require stitches and can be very sore but are unlikely to cause long-term problems.
- **Third-degree tears.** These extend downwards from the vaginal wall and perineum and affect the muscle that controls the anus (the anal sphincter). Along with fourth-degree tears (below), these are also called obstetric anal sphincter injuries (OASI) and together they affect around 3 per cent of women having vaginal births. The anal sphincter is important for anal continence (preventing the leakage of gas and faeces) and a tear like this would need to be repaired in an operating theatre.

- **Fourth-degree tears.** Similar to a third-degree tear, but this extends further into the lining of the anus or rectum. Like a third-degree tear, this would also need to be repaired in an operating theatre. Usually, ongoing physiotherapy and assessment would be needed to ensure long-term damage is reduced.

Episiotomy

An episiotomy is a cut made by your midwife or doctor into the perineum and vaginal wall to make more room for your baby. This is usually repaired using dissolvable stitches after labour.

Things to consider

You may well be sore for some time after a vaginal delivery, due to bruising, stretching of the pelvic floor and potential tears or episiotomies.

First off, you might want to consider how you can be most comfortable when seated. Sitting on a ring-shaped or 'doughnut' cushion can help to relieve the pressure on any bruised bits, or you could try some side-lying instead.

Pelvic floor exercises can be performed as soon as you feel ready (and if there is no catheter in place) and can really help to speed up recovery by increasing the circulation of blood to the area and taking the pressure off of any tears and surrounding tissue. You may find that at first you don't 'feel' much happening, as the muscles will be stretched and have lost some of their tone. Don't panic – this is normal. But with stimulation (in the form of pelvic floor exercises) the muscles should start to gain strength and tone again soon. It'll take time and effort, but it's worth it.

As you make your way through the exercises that follow, consider using pillows and props to ensure you are comfortable, no matter what you're doing. I might suggest you start an exercise seated, but if it isn't comfortable, don't push through the pain – there's always an alternative position.

It's important that you have read and understood the section on pressure management on p. 174, as this will help when you start to reintroduce core work. Your pelvic floor could be considered a 'path of least resistance' here (see p. 175), so you would want to make sure you are aware of how to manage the pressure you create, and when to regress an exercise.

It's important that you relay any concerns you may have, regarding pain or incontinence, to your GP and ask for a pelvic health referral if something isn't right. You know your body better than anyone.

Caesarean delivery – what happens to your body?

So you've had a Caesarean. How are you feeling? I know so many women, myself included, who have had elective Caesareans that were gentle and calm, and their recoveries were fast and simple. I also know many women, again myself included, who had emergency or unplanned Caesareans that were traumatic and painful, with slower recoveries and all sorts of emotions they didn't expect. It's also possible that you fit into both of those two categories in some way. As always, it's important to acknowledge that no two births are the same and no two Caesareans are the same, and, once again, I hope that those of you who need support are able to access it.

When it comes to a Caesarean birth, regardless of the circumstances, there's no getting away from the fact that it is major abdominal surgery. And although there is no formal hierarchy of sh*t births, there is almost always going to be a longer recovery time for someone who had a Caesarean compared to someone who had a smooth vaginal birth.

Movement is slightly limited after a Caesarean, due to stitches and potential pain, and you do need to allow your tissue time to heal. This can be straightforward, but I want to be honest – you may be starting certain movements and exercises a little later than someone with a different birth experience. The moral of the story here is that you must try not to compare yourself to others. You need to move at a pace that works for you and where you are at in your postnatal journey.

I'm not going to go into huge depth about what Caesarean surgery entails, but I will touch on what it might mean for your recovery. If you are still at a stage where you can't think about your surgery, can't bear to look at your scar or you are having flashbacks, this may not be the time to read this section. Please do consider your mental health when reading the next page or so.

The actual surgery

Around one in four pregnant women in the UK has a Caesarean section[3], whether elective (planned ahead of time) or unplanned (emergency), with most falling into the second category.

During a Caesarean delivery, your surgeon will cut through six layers of tissue to get to your uterus, and hence your baby. The cuts are generally between 10 and 20cm long, just below your bikini line, and usually in a horizontal line, although some will be vertical.

A worry for many women is that their abdominals are cut through and damaged in the procedure. However, the rectus abdominis muscles are separated to get to the baby and are not cut (except in very rare circumstances). This means that any core weakness you experience postnatally is usually due to deconditioning, rather than damage.

After the surgery

Women often feel very tender and fragile after a Caesarean, and this can mean they hunch over and avoid moving for fear of damaging their scar. This is totally understandable, and I felt exactly this way after my first; however, a little bit of movement is important when ready. Your stitches are strong and you need to get up and move around to reduce your risk of blood clots. Scar tissue also needs to be able to move and glide, so sticking to one very specific huddled position isn't advisable, I'm afraid.

Things to consider

You will likely feel sore (do stay on top of your pain relief, as it can be hard to 'play catch up' if you come off it too quickly) and, as mentioned, nervous to move at first, but it is important that you do. Walking, when you feel ready, is helpful (plus it's low impact), but I wouldn't carry the baby in a baby carrier in the first few weeks, as this can put unnecessary downward pressure on your scar area.

When it comes to your recovery phase movements or any recommended exercises, please ensure you are comfortable, and if something doesn't feel right, stop or change positions. Your scar should start to feel less tender after a few weeks, but for some it may take longer. I have found that, as with my own experience, Bump Plan members who had elective Caesareans have recovered slightly quicker (or felt less fragile quicker) than those who had emergency ones, but again, this is not a hard-and-fast rule.

It's also worth remembering that some of us will have gone into surgery after days of attempting a vaginal labour. We may be exhausted after delivery because we were awake (and essentially running a marathon) pre-surgery. Again, you need to consider this when thinking about recovery times.

As with vaginal births, it's important that you have read and understood the section on pressure management on p. 174. When you start to reintroduce core work, your scar could be considered a 'path of least resistance' (see p. 175), so you should be aware of how to manage the pressure you create and when to regress an exercise.

And please note the following warning signs – if you notice any of these, you must contact your midwife or GP immediately, as they could be a sign of a blood clot or infection:

- Severe pain
- Leaking urine
- Pain when peeing
- Heavy vaginal bleeding
- Your wound becomes more red, painful and swollen
- A discharge of pus or foul-smelling fluid from your wound
- A cough or shortness of breath
- Swelling or pain in your lower leg

A note on all births

The path back to movement will look *similar*, no matter how you gave birth. All women will be aiming to get back to the same guidelines (which we'll discuss in a moment) and might hit the same speed bumps. But there is no denying that how your body feels, and the recovery timelines you can expect, will probably look different depending on how you gave birth. You may find that you need to use props to be comfortable during certain movements; you might need to regress an exercise that simply feels a little too advanced; and it could be that Tracy down the pub is 'ahead' of you with regards to postnatal recovery. All of this is fine and normal and part of the beauty that we are all different. Please focus on *your* progress alone, without comparing yourself to anyone else, and I promise you'll get back to the movement you love with time.

The guidelines

Thankfully, guidelines on postnatal physical activity do exist, again thanks to the CMOs. If you've done your reading in Part 1, you'll recognise them, so here goes. The official Chief Medical Officers' physical activity guidelines for women after childbirth (birth to 12 months) are . . . '*to aim for at least 150 minutes of moderate intensity activity every week*'.

Oh my gosh. That guideline again! The same as pre-conception, the same as pregnancy and now the same postnatally. And again, this is because we want everyone to eventually get back to this magic number (at least 150 minutes) because there are so many proven physical and mental health benefits at this level.

However, the key thing here is to aim towards meeting the guidelines gradually. Please do not expect that you'll be hitting these numbers the day after you give birth.

The official, proven benefits to *building back up* to the guidelines are as follows:

- It helps provide some time for yourself – some 'me-time' – and although this can be hard, it can really help to reduce worries and depression.
- It can help with a return to pre-pregnancy weight. Now personally, I stay away from discussing women's weight, and I am not an instructor that sells weight loss as a service, but medically this is listed as a benefit by the CMOs.
- It improves tummy-muscle tone and strength – training your core effectively will help you to regain your core strength. Remember, if you don't use it, you lose it.
- It improves fitness, sleep and mood – I mean who wouldn't want these benefits? I can't guarantee that you'll get *more* sleep, but it does help with sleep quality, which can be so beneficial in the early days when sleep isn't your most available commodity.

The guidelines also stress that it's worth starting daily pelvic floor exercises as soon as you feel able to, and that you build back up to muscle strengthening activities twice per week. You'll find instructions for both later on in Part 3.

If you were already active during pregnancy, keep going; however, if you were previously inactive, start gradually and build up. Much of the advice here requires an element of listening to your body. I know that can be tricky at times (especially when your mind is so focused on your new little one), but I genuinely believe that exercise can really help you to listen to how your body feels, and what it is telling you.

Before we jump into the postpartum 'phases', however, there are a couple of common issues that crop up postnatally that it's helpful to be aware of.

Diastasis

We talked in Parts 1 and 2 about diastasis recti (head to p. 167 to swot up), which is thought to be a functional effect of pregnancy. Studies suggest that up to 100 per cent of women will have some form of diastasis by the time they give birth[4], and that for two thirds, it will resolve itself postnatally with no issues.[5] For the final third of women, a lot can be done with postnatal core rehab to improve function, and this will feature heavily in the Bump Plan postnatal exercises.

Postnatally, diastasis can leave you with a pendular appearance in the tummy area – so side on, the tummy can look distended (sadly, the term 'mum tum' is often used here). This is because the linea alba has stretched and thinned and hasn't yet regained its pull on the abdominal wall, therefore affecting the appearance of this area.

This might be an issue for some from an aesthetic point of view (and I don't want to discredit that at all here), but you can still be functional, strong and fit, with a diastasis. You can still do core work, and it doesn't mean you'll never be able to do a plank again. What it does usually mean is that you'll need to have a little more awareness of pressure management (see p. 174), and you'll need to be more mindful of which exercises you perform and *how*.

If you think you may have a diastasis, seek an assessment from a health professional (usually a physiotherapist). To diagnose you, they usually need to perform an ultrasound. You can ask your GP for a referral to a physiotherapist – but know that the exercises I list in this book could help, and I take diastasis into consideration throughout.

Prolapse

Prolapse, or pelvic organ prolapse (POP), is described as a vaginal change, where a pelvic organ – which may be the bladder, bowel, rectum or uterus – moves downwards in the vagina causing the sensation of 'something coming down' or a feeling of vaginal heaviness.[6] Prolapse is very common, with one in three women who have had children being affected by it.

A prolapse is more likely when the pelvic floor muscles and the ligaments that support them are weakened and struggle to do their job. This then allows the weight of one (or more) of the pelvic organs to descend into the vagina.

During pregnancy, the weight of the growing uterus puts a lot of pressure on the pelvic floor muscles, and hormones encourage a relaxation of the ligaments of the pelvis. This, particularly combined with a vaginal birth, is the most common factor for prolapse. If you have had significant tearing, an episiotomy or a forceps delivery, you are also more likely to experience a prolapse.

For some women, a prolapse will be painless and not bother them, while for others, it will be severe and affect their lives in various ways. A prolapse can also vary from day to day and even at different times of the day or after certain activities (such as standing for long periods of time, or after emptying your bowels).

If you are concerned you may have a prolapse, please ask your GP to refer you to a pelvic health physiotherapist (they are gods), so they can assess you and give you specific guidance.

There are various treatment methods, and a few of them are covered in general postnatal rehab, which is helpful, so if you know you have a prolapse, the exercises in the recovery phase and phase 1 should really help. Strengthening the pelvic floor muscles, for many, will help bring back the support needed for the pelvic organs. This, plus an awareness of pressure management (which you can read up on p. 174), should really help you to manage your symptoms.

When it comes to reintroducing impact into your training (which is where phase 2 comes in), this usually requires some trial and error. Hopefully, by this stage you'll be under the guidance of a pelvic health physiotherapist, and you'll have been working on your pelvic floor exercises and understand pressure management. You may also be using a pessary and working with your physio to build impact into your training. It's particularly important that in phase 2 you really listen to your body and see how impact feels for you. If you find it makes your symptoms worse, it's usually a sign that you need to reduce it.

Overall, though, as with diastasis, a prolapse doesn't mean that you can't get back to *you* again and doing the things you love. It may just take a little time, a fair amount of effort and some awareness and education of what is happening in your body to resume certain movements or forms of training. You've got this (but please do push for support from a pelvic health physio).

So that covers some of the things you might need to know ahead of getting your body moving postnatally. Now let's get stuck in.

How to use Part 3

My belief is that once you've had a baby, you are always 'postnatal'. Your body – and your life – changes immeasurably, and this is life-long. I say this because it's not just those of you who are 2 weeks post-labour who can benefit from (or are justified to do) 'postnatal training'. You may be 9 months postpartum or 18 months, and not see yourself as specifically 'postnatal', but you can still benefit from starting at phase 1 if you have yet to reintroduce any physical activity into your life. Be realistic and honest about where you *actually are* in your postnatal journey and start there.

It's impossible to put definitive time frames on postnatal recovery, as every fertility journey, pregnancy, labour and post-natal situation is different. Two women could outwardly seem to have had the same experiences, but their bodies may have reacted in very different ways. For this reason, I won't be specify-ing time frames for this part of the book. Instead, I will give you an indication as to who each phase might be best suited to.

I will talk you through how to gradually progress back to the movement you love, starting with the recovery phase (for very early days post-labour), through postnatal phase 1 (where we reintroduce more dynamic core work) and postnatal phase 2 (where we introduce impact). For each phase, I will explain who should use it and what we'll be covering, so you can assess where you think you may need to start. I'll also go into what you need to know in order to move your body safely in each phase, and list the exercises I would love you to introduce into your training. I'll also give you information at the end of each phase about when it's time to 'move on' to the next one.

As you progress through the postnatal phases of this book, it's important to listen to your body and assess how your pelvic floor copes with an increase in core load or impact. It may be that you choose to skip back to a previous phase if the next one doesn't feel right yet. You must learn to drop the ego, take your time and be kind to yourself. This is a marathon, not a sprint, so please do take one phase at a time.

Remember that postnatal recovery may not always be linear. You may feel fantastic for a few weeks if you have plenty of childcare and, perhaps, a sleepy baby, so that you find time to move your body a lot. And then there may be weeks when you get less sleep, have zero childcare or just generally feel wiped out, and you can't manage as much. For some reason, we can really beat ourselves up when it comes to fitness, but please don't. This is life.

Recovery phase

The recovery phase is designed for those who have just given birth, are maybe yet to have their 6-week check-up, still feel a little tender or apprehensive but want to start laying the foundations of movement. This might be when you are 1 week post-vaginal birth or maybe 3 weeks post-Caesarean section – as always, it really will vary from person to person. If you try some of the movements or activities in this section and they just don't feel right (i.e. if something feels too difficult, painful or you find yourself falling into poor technique to manage it), remember that you can always wait a little longer, and come back to it when you're ready.

What will we be covering?

This phase aims to get your body moving gently, rehabilitate your muscles and start to give your body the awareness it needs ahead of any higher-level movement in phases 1 and 2. Imagine it as almost waking your body up, while also easing some of the aches and pains that can linger from labour and those first few days and weeks of parenting.

This section comprises the pelvic floor routine, the breathwork routine, the deep-core-activation routine and the gentle stretching routine. You don't have to do them in sequence, at specific times, but as you begin recovery, doing some of them often will really help to lay the foundations for phases 1 and 2.

There are no set 'routines' in the recovery phase but, in an ideal world, you would do the pelvic floor routine daily, 2–3 times. You could do a few pelvic floor holds each time you feed your baby if you find it helpful to have a reminder to nudge you along. The breathwork, deep-core-activation and gentle stretching routines could/should be done daily, if time allows – but what matters most is that they are performed well. Quality over quantity is really important, and I'm sure you're fast discovering how demanding those first few weeks can be, so do be kind to yourself if you're struggling to fit them in as often as you'd like.

What do I need to know?

It can really help to spend some time reviewing the information on the pelvic floor (see p. 51), breathwork (see p. 126) and the abdominals (see p. 45) ahead of the movements in this section, so that you really understand what is being asked of you, and what is going on beneath the skin. This awareness will help you to perform the movements safely and effectively and give you an appreciation of just what your body has been through and achieved in the last 9+ months.

Your exercises: recovery phase

So without further ado, let's get into the exercises you'll be working through during the recovery phase. Remember, how long this phase lasts is completely up to you.

Your pelvic floor routine

Understandably, the pelvic floor can feel a little 'different' after having a baby. And not just for those who've experienced a vaginal birth – because you've all carried an increasingly large weight around with you for the last 9 months. Re-finding the pelvic floor is important and, over time, it'll get easier to feel/activate. Aim to do these 3 times a day:

1. Start in a position that is comfortable for you. That might be seated or side-lying, but standing would be one of the hardest positions, so I wouldn't advise that just yet. Close your eyes (if possible) and focus on your breath.
2. Inhale and, as you exhale, think about squeezing and lifting the pelvic floor muscles, and hold. Hold for as long as you can (up to 8–10 seconds) and then relax. Aim for 10 long holds.
3. Now try 10 fast pulses, where you squeeze and release rapidly.

TIP: Don't worry if your holds don't feel very long at first. It should feel challenging, so do push yourself here, and your holds should get longer the more you practise them. Use a visualisation that works for you: this might be imagining picking up blueberries with your vagina or sucking a smoothie through a straw – whatever resonates with you and encourages both a squeezing of the pelvic holes (urethra, vagina and anus) and a lifting.

REGRESSION: you want the pelvic floor muscles to feel tired by the end of this, so try not to make it too easy, but you can start with shorter holds or fewer repetitions, if that helps, and then build up over time.

PROGRESSION: as mentioned, standing is one the hardest positions to practise your pelvic floor exercises in, so you could build up to that for a challenge when ready.

Your breathwork routine

During pregnancy, your breathing technique can really change, due to alterations in intra-abdominal pressure and your uterus growing up towards your main breathing muscle – the diaphragm (see pp. 124–125). Postnatally, it can be beneficial to practise effective, diaphragmatic breathing to help strengthen that muscle. It also has the effect of naturally stimulating the pelvic floor and the abdominal muscles. Oh, and it's also been shown to calm us down and reduce blood pressure, which I'm sure, as parents, we all need. (See also p. 126 for more about the concept and benefits of diaphragmatic breathing.)

Note: this is the same technique as the breathwork routine on p. 178 in Part 2.

1. Make sure you are sitting, lying or standing in a comfortable position. (Personally, I like doing this seated or side-lying.)
2. Begin by inhaling through your nose and exhaling through your mouth. Get this circular pattern of breathing started first.
3. With each inhale, start to visualise the diaphragm contracting and sucking air into the lungs, until there is no space left.
4. On the exhale, imagine the diaphragm relaxing and all the air from the lungs being emptied out; keep exhaling, until there is no more air left in the lungs.
5. Start to notice how the core expands on the inhale and relaxes as you exhale.
6. As you inhale, imagine the ribcage expanding in all directions (out to the sides, front and back), and on the exhale, notice it contracting back inwards.
7. Continue for up to 5 minutes, then relax and breathe in your normal fashion.

TIP: It's easy to overthink diaphragmatic breathing – but it doesn't have to be perfect. Simply spending some time listening to your breath and trying to breathe a little deeper – all of which is encouraging you to be mindful – can make a huge difference.

There are no regressions or progressions here. Just practise when you can, or when you feel your emotions may need calming down.

Your deep core activation routine

You may recognise this as the Abdominal Hollowing exercise from the TTC chapter of Part 1. It's also helpful postnatally because it stimulates the transversus abdominis, which stretches during pregnancy. Abdominal hollowing is a simple, effective exercise to target that muscle.

When you think about the 'deep core', it can feel elusive postnatally. I remember feeling really soft, weak and almost as if I had no abdominals left at all. But I promise it won't feel like that for ever and you will start to feel your core strength return with time and stimulation. And this routine will help.

1. Start in a comfortable position (seated, side-lying, standing) and with your hands resting on your tummy near your belly button.
2. Inhale and then, as you exhale, think about lifting up your pelvic floor and activating your transversus abdominis. As you inhale, relax.
3. Repeat 6–8 times.

TIP: There are a few ways you can imagine activating your transversus abdominis: you could imagine that you are drawing in your tummy slightly, that someone is tightening up a corset around your waist or that you are trying to do up a pair of tight jeans. What you should feel under your hands is a slight inward pulling of your tummy. It's not aggressive, and you should still be able to breathe. There should also be no pain!

REGRESSION: start with just the pelvic floor lift or just the transversus abdominis activation, then build up to doing both together.

PROGRESSION: add a 10-second hold at the end but ensure you can still breathe or talk while holding.

Your gentle stretching routine

Life with a newborn can be pretty sedentary, and you may find that you are stuck in the same position all day (sat down, hunched over, shoulders rounded). This can leave you feeling stiff, with an achy neck, and a deep desire to be in any position other than that. So really, what you are attempting here is to simply move your body into the opposite position to the one that it is in all day.

Seated side bend

In a comfortable seated position, with hands either in prayer position or fingers to your temples, gently bend your spine to the left side, feeling an enjoyable stretch down the right side of your waist. Hold for a few deep breaths, and then come back to neutral. Repeat on the other side and do four side bends on each side.

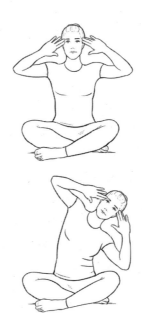

Seated rotation

In a comfortable seated position, with hands either in prayer position or fingers to your temples, rotate your upper body to the left. Hold for a few deep breaths, and then come back to neutral. Repeat on the other side and do four rotations on each side.

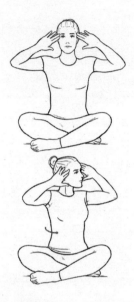

Seated thoracic extension

In a comfortable seated position, with hands either in prayer position or fingers to your temples, inhale and start to lift your eyes and chest upwards to the ceiling, lengthening out your spine and extending your thoracic spine (your upper back). Stay in this position for a few deep breaths, and then come back to neutral. Repeat 4 times.

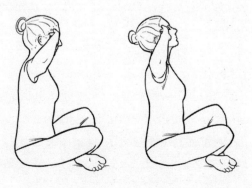

How to cope with birth trauma

by Illy Morrison, midwife, birth debrief facilitator and mother of two

If you had a difficult birth, you may be experiencing signs of birth trauma. This information is included to help you navigate traumatic feelings relating to your baby's birth, but if you need further support, contact your GP, the Birth Trauma Association or your local support group.

What is birth trauma?

Birth trauma is a term often used to describe PTSD (post-traumatic stress disorder) associated with the perinatal period (from the beginning of pregnancy up to a year after giving birth), but importantly, it is used in regard to those who might have *some* symptoms of PTSD but not full-blown PTSD. These symptoms include flashbacks, nightmares and intrusive thoughts, hypervigilance (feeling on high alert all the time) and finding difficulty in seeing or going past the place where the trauma took place. You may have other symptoms as well, including low mood, feelings of guilt and shame. Trauma is not something that happens to you, but more the way your body responds to an event that has taken place.

Why might someone suffer from birth trauma?

There are many who will suffer from trauma for a magnitude of reasons, from physical complications such as major blood loss, the length of labour (both long and short) or a clinical birth intervention (such as induction of labour, forceps, ventouse or C-section) and stillbirth. Some other reasons might be not being listened to, not being heard, not being supported or being ignored. Perhaps, you have been spoken to poorly by professionals, or your partner hasn't supported you. For some, it could be a postnatal experience, such as the baby being admitted to special care or you, the mother, being admitted to high-risk care.

Previous trauma such as sexual assault or childhood trauma may also be the reason behind birth trauma. Many things may be behind it, and it is important that I don't dictate the cause because it is so deeply personal. Remember, it was traumatic if it felt traumatic to you.

What are the treatment options?

There are numerous options for initially addressing birth trauma. Most hospital trusts offer a birth-reflection service – this is more often than not the opportunity to go through your clinical notes and to understand what happened and ask any questions you may have. There are concerns about this service, however – the most important being that there is a lack of impartiality and the risk of defensive practice (where the facilitator may be overprotective of their colleague). However, as practitioners become more trauma aware, there is hope that this is reducing.

You can also access a private birth-reflection service which may be more comfortable due to the impartiality and the fact that you will not have to return to or be in close proximity to the place or the people associated with the trauma.

The most commonly offered treatment option for birth trauma is cognitive behavioural therapy (CBT), which works by changing thought patterns and finding coping mechanisms for the trauma and the symptoms.

Eye movement desensitisation and reprocessing (EMDR) is a more specialised treatment option for birth trauma and PTSD. It is used to alleviate any distress that comes with memories of the traumatic event. The patient is helped to access the memories and adapt them in a way that brings them some form of resolution.

Talking therapy with a qualified birth-trauma therapist is another option. If this is something you are interested in, I would most certainly advise seeking someone who is qualified in birth trauma in order to facilitate healing.

How might birth trauma affect future pregnancies?

For many, subsequent pregnancies can throw up issues of previous trauma, despite work having being done to overcome it. This is normal – to be expected, even. You have the option of speaking to your midwife about it and seeing what plans you can put in place – both clinically and emotionally. Making a birth plan that is applicable to your lived experience is important. You know the challenges that you faced last time, so what can you control next time, what can you mitigate and how? These are the questions to ask both yourself, your birth support and your care team next time around.

Postnatal phase 1

Phase 1 is the next step of the postnatal journey and is ideal for those who have worked through the recovery phase, feel ready to move their bodies more and whose scars are healing well. Some women may join this phase 6 weeks post-vaginal birth, others might join it 10 weeks post-Caesarean, but we are all different, so please listen to your body, only do what feels right for you and consult your GP if you're unsure.

What will we be covering?

In postnatal phase 1, I'm going to start introducing some dynamic abdominal work into your training and you'll assess how you are managing the pressure created in these exercises and how your core copes with the extra demand. There will be some loaded flexion-based exercises (these require you to use your abdominals to flex the spine, as in an abdominal crunch/sit-up; they are usually, but not always, done lying on your back) and also some dynamic standing work. All the exercises in this phase are strength based; in postnatal phase 2, you'll build on them, as well as introducing some impact and cardiovascular exercise.

Because there's no cardiovascular element in this phase, you don't need to warm up or cool down pre- or post-exercise. If you were about to perform cardiovascular exercises, you would want to gradually increase your heart rate beforehand, but because phase 1 is purely focused on musculoskeletal strength, there is no strong benefit to completing a warm-up or cool-down (gradually bringing the heart rate back to pre-exercise levels).

Now you'll notice with these moves that each, in fact, is two exercises in one, starting with the easiest version, for those who are just entering phase 1, and then a more advanced option to build up to. This way, you are constantly being challenged (which is required for strength improvements), and once you have mastered the more advanced version, you're probably ready for phase 2.

What do I need to know?

There can be a lot of confusion around reintroducing abdominal work postnatally. Some of this stems from a lack of clarity about diastasis, and some from a lack of information on where best to start with postnatal core training. I'd recommend taking another look at Antony Lo's advice on diastasis (see p. 167) before reading on.

For those who believe they may still have a diastasis, there can be a lot of fear of movement, but this needn't be the case. We all need strong cores, and we can't just avoid core work for fear of making a diastasis worse (plus, it's very unlikely that would happen, anyway). My advice is to adopt the same strategies that I recommended during pregnancy (it's thought we all have some level of diastasis by the time we give birth), which means reading up on pressure management again (see p. 174) and understanding how to apply this in the core.

During each exercise, I want you to be aware of how it makes your body feel. When you move your body, you create a change in intra-abdominal pressure, and need to be slightly aware of how that is managed by you. If you feel a lot of pressure down your tummy's midline (your linea alba) and see hard-doming (where it looks like a big Toblerone and feels hard when you touch it), you might want to consider making the exercise a little easier, using one of the regressions, while your tissues are trying to remodel and adapt.

The same goes for your pelvic floor – if you feel lots of pressure down there during an exercise, or you leak urine, faeces or wind, it may be worth regressing the move, until it is manageable, and then build up gradually.

If you have any scars (Caesarean or vaginal), please also be mindful of how they feel during these movements. You really need to tap into that mind–body connection (simply listening to and being aware of your body and how it feels) to ensure you are allowing your scars the opportunity to heal, while also building strength to support them.

This may take some time to get used to, and I know it can be so much harder to concentrate when there's a little one near by who needs your attention, too. Try to carve out some time to focus on the exercises you do practise, though, so you can be sure of good technique, and be mindful of how they make your body feel.

Alongside these strengthening exercises, please also feel free to add in any low-impact cardiovascular exercise that feels safe and comfortable for your body. Walking is one of the best things you could include here, as it's low impact, easy, free and you can bring your baby with you (if you want to). You can start with very short walks, and gradually build up as you feel able to do so. Remember, you are aiming to get back up to the CMOs' postnatal physical activity guidelines, so please do refer to those if you need a refresher (see p. 254).

Your exercises: phase 1

Now it's time to give your postnatal phase 1 exercises a try. You'll find sample routines at the end of this section.

Do remember that for each exercise there is an easier option to start with, and a progression to build up to as you get stronger and feel ready.

Pelvic tilts to hip rolls

Pelvic tilts are a great way to get the abdominals and lower back muscles switched on (as they create the movement) but they can also feel great from a mobility point of view. You can do them in other positions, too (such as standing, kneeling and on hands and knees). I like doing them supine (on my back), so I can feel the feedback from the floor as I move. Progressing to hip rolls can help to fire up the glutes (which can lengthen and lose tone during pregnancy) and gets even more of the spine moving and articulating, which should feel great.

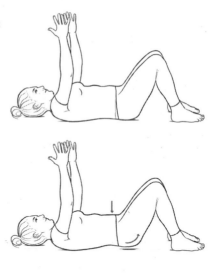

1. Start lying on your back, knees bent, feet and knees hip-width apart. You want to aim for a neutral spine, which, in this position, means the hip and pubic bones are roughly level (or imagine there's a blueberry under your lower back that you don't want to squash).
2. Inhale and, as you exhale, visualise bringing your hip bones and ribcage closer together, and the lower back pressing gently into the floor.
3. Inhale to return the pelvis to neutral.
4. Repeat 10–12 times.

Progression – hip rolls

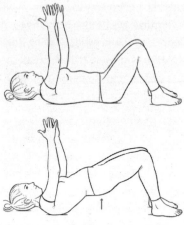

1. Start in the same position.
2. Inhale to press the lower back towards the mat and then, as you exhale, start to lift the hips up using your glutes and peel the spine away from the floor, one vertebra at a time, until you have created a diagonal line from the base of the ribcage to the knees.
3. Inhale to stay, then exhale to slowly peel back down through the spine, a vertebra at a time, to return to the start position.
4. Repeat 8–10 times.

TIP: For both exercises, think about the abdominals shortening to help create the initial pelvic tilt (rather than just clenching your bum cheeks). When progressing to hip rolls, you want the glutes to push the hips up towards the ceiling (and create hip extension), so press your feet into the ground and drive your knees forwards, over your toes, as you lift your hips.

Zips to knee lifts

Zips are a great way to reconnect with your pelvic floor and transversus abdominis, while also learning to manage core pressure. By lifting your pelvic floor first, you prevent bearing down on it when you activate the transversus abdominis muscle (which creates more core pressure). Adding in the knee lifts will help to challenge this skill, and develop core endurance, while also helping to build strength and endurance in the shoulders.

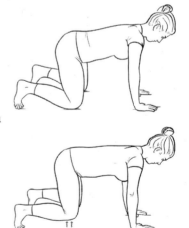

1. Start on hands and knees, with a nice, neutral spine and the core relaxed.
2. Visualise a zip running from the tailbone, past your pubic bone, past your belly button and up to your sternum (the middle of your ribcage).
3. Start with the zip 'unzipped'. Inhale and then, as you exhale, imagine 'zipping up' from tailbone to sternum.
4. Inhale to unzip, back from sternum to tailbone.
5. Repeat 10–12 times.

Progression – knee lifts

1. Start in the same position.
2. Zip up as above, and then maintain this feeling of core engagement.
3. Inhale to prepare and then, as you exhale, start to slowly lift the knees up away from the floor a few centimetres to hover.
4. Inhale to release with control.
5. Repeat 6–8 times.

TIP: Really think about creating an even contraction of the core when you zip up, rather than just sucking your belly button to your spine (which we don't want). It can help to visualise the corset effect of the transversus abdominis muscle that we have discussed previously (see p. 158). When you add in the knee lifts, monitor how your core reacts – ideally, you want the abdominals to stay looking similar as the knees lift, rather than suddenly popping out.

Head unweighting to ab prep

Head unweighting is a great exercise for priming the neck and core for flexion again. You have no doubt spent the last 7+ months skipping this type of movement (think abdominal crunches), so there will be some deconditioning here. Head unweighting helps you to gradually reintroduce this challenge and learn good technique, too. And progressing to ab prep will then allow you to test out and develop this technique.

1. Start lying on your back, knees bent, feet hip-width apart, arms relaxed by your sides. Try to find a neutral spine and pelvis, keeping your eyeline directly up towards the ceiling.
2. Inhale to prepare and then, as you exhale, imagine you have a blueberry under your head that you don't want to squash. You are essentially making your head as light as possible ('unweighting') without actually lifting it off the floor.
3. Inhale to release back to the start.
4. Repeat 8–10 times.

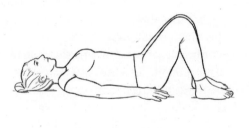

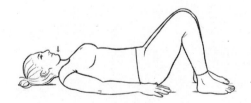

Progression – ab prep

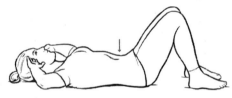

1. Start in the same position, but bring your fingers to your temples, elbows wide.
2. Inhale and nod your head slightly, as though giving yourself a little double chin.
3. As you exhale, start to lift the head and shoulders away from the floor, flexing your upper spine, and drawing your ribcage down towards your hip bones.

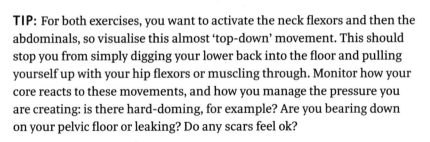

4. Inhale to stay here, and exhale to lower back down with control. Repeat 8–10 times.

TIP: For both exercises, you want to activate the neck flexors and then the abdominals, so visualise this almost 'top-down' movement. This should stop you from simply digging your lower back into the floor and pulling yourself up with your hip flexors or muscling through. Monitor how your core reacts to these movements, and how you manage the pressure you are creating: is there hard-doming, for example? Are you bearing down on your pelvic floor or leaking? Do any scars feel ok?

Knee folds to single leg extensions

Often, new clients will start training with me thinking that the only way to strengthen their core is with loaded flexion – i.e. crunches. However, in these two exercises you'll be developing core strength without having to lift your head off the mat at all. Leaving the head down on the mat, can help to prevent neck tension creeping in while you rebuild core strength, instead using the weight of the legs as resistance for the core.

1. Start lying on your back, knees bent, feet hip-width apart, arms relaxed by your sides. Try to find a neutral spine and pelvis and keep your eyeline directly up towards the ceiling – maintain this as you move.
2. Inhale to prepare and, as you exhale, slowly float the left leg up to a tabletop position.
3. Inhale to slowly lower it back to the floor.
4. Repeat with the right leg.
5. Now you can continue in this way (lifting one leg only at a time) or you can lift the left leg, then also the right leg, then lower the left leg, then lower the right leg (so at some point both legs are in tabletop position).
6. Continue for 60–90 seconds.

Progression – single leg extensions

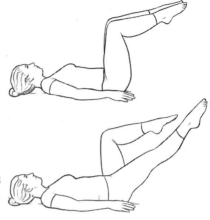

1. Start as above, but with both legs already in a tabletop position.
2. Inhale to prepare and, as you exhale, slowly extend your right leg out towards the end of your mat, only as low as you can keep your pelvis still.
3. Inhale to return it to the start.
4. Repeat with the left leg.
5. Repeat 8–10 times per leg.

TIP: It's *really* important here – for both exercises – that the rest of the body stays still. This means keeping the pelvis stable using the muscles of the core, rather than rocking back and forth as your legs move. I like to rest my hands on my pelvis or abdominal area to feel for any movement there. If you are struggling with this, reduce the range of movement or slow the movement down, and try activating the core a little more (use your 'zip' technique here, if it helps – see p. 158).

Mini hip hinges to full hip hinges

I know I'm like a broken record, but hip hinges are part of everyday life, particularly for parents, and we cannot (and should not) avoid them. Every time you look down into your baby's cot, every time you run their bath or change their nappy, every time you wipe their nose you are in a hip hinge position (and if you're not, you should be). So you'd better learn good technique, and build endurance to cope with this!

1. Start in a neutral standing position, with your hands in prayer position at your chest.
2. As you inhale, start to hinge at your hips, almost as though you are bowing, just enough to feel the beginnings of a little stretch up the back of the body.
3. Exhale to push down into your feet and bring yourself back to your start position.
4. Repeat 8–10 times.

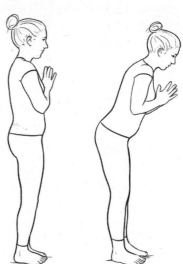

Progression – full hip hinges

The only difference here is you are finding your maximum range/progressing this to a *full* hip hinge.

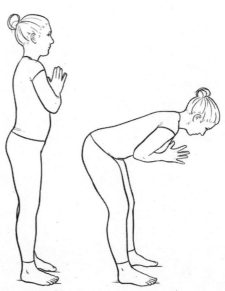

1. When you hinge/bow this time, go as far as you can manage. Eventually, you'll hit a point where you can go no further, and you feel a stretch up the back of the body that holds you back.

2. Once you hit this point, exhale to press the feet into the floor and bring yourself back to your start position.
3. Repeat 8–10 times.

TIP: Aim to keep the movement within the hip joint only, so no other joints really change here. Your spine should stay neutral as you move (so no hunching over or overextending your spine and back bending) and your knees stay soft (rather than bending as you hinge). This is simply flexion and extension of the hips, so direct your mind–body connection to that area.

Static baby lunges to full lunges

Lunges are another really functional movement that's important to practise outside of everyday life. You are lunging when you climb stairs, when you lunge to catch your child when they fall, when you pick up toys from the floor. Good technique and endurance are a must as a parent.

1. Start in a nice, neutral standing position, hands in prayer position at your chest.

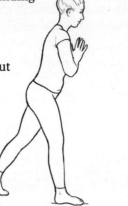
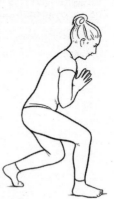

2. Step your right foot forwards, as if you're about to walk off your mat, keeping the feet roughly hip-width apart (rather than standing on an imaginary tightrope) and rise up on to the ball of your left foot. This is your lunge start position and the hips should be pointing forwards. Hip hinge forwards a little to ensure you still have a neutral spine here.
3. Inhale to bend both knees, lowering your body down towards the floor.
4. Exhale to push into the feet and bring yourself back to standing.
5. Repeat 8–10 times, then swap legs.

Progression – full lunges

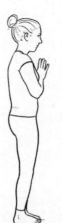
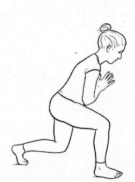

1. Start in a nice, neutral standing position, hands in prayer position at your chest.
2. Step the right foot forwards as if you're about to walk off your mat, hip hinge forwards slightly to maintain a neutral spine and bend both knees, bringing your body down towards the floor.

3. Exhale to press through your right foot, push yourself back to standing and bring the right foot back in to your start position.
4. Repeat 8–10 times, then swap legs.

TIP: You'll need to play around with how far forwards you step your front foot here, as you want to feel stable and not step so far that you feel wobbly; but also, you don't want to feel limited as to how low you can lunge. The aim is to bend both knees in the lunges, but almost favour the front leg to help get you back to standing. Keep both hips pointing forwards as you lunge and aim for a neutral spine (i.e. don't feel you have to keep looking ahead as you lunge, as this can cause you to lean back as you lunge down).

Mini squats (to sitting) to full squats

Squats are another basic movement pattern that you will be including in your life already, but usually with a baby/car-seat/heavy-bag situation going on that means your technique is wonky, loaded more on one side or simply performed without much awareness (totally fair enough!). Here's an opportunity to practise your squat technique without all the baggage, and with an appreciation of good technique.

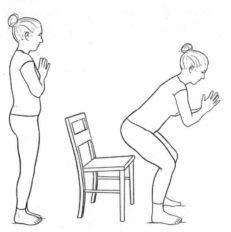

1. Start in a nice, neutral standing position, hands in prayer position at your chest and a chair placed behind you.
2. Inhale and start to bend your knees, hip hinging forwards as you do so, and imagine you are about to place your bum slowly down on the chair behind you. (It's up to you how far you go, but I would advise that you start small and eventually build up to actually tapping your bum on the chair lightly.)
3. As you exhale, push down into your feet and come back up to your start position.
4. Repeat 8–10 times.

Progression – full squats

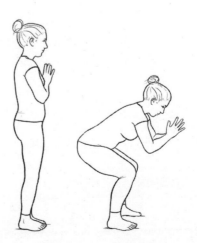

This is the same as the above exercise but remove the chair this time.

1. Use the same technique, and still imagine that you are lowering down on to a chair – but see if you can go a little lower into your squat, despite losing the safety of the chair.
2. Repeat 10–12 times.

TIP: I often see squats being performed incorrectly – people only bending at their hips and not bending their knees too, or simply rounding their backs, focusing on touching their toes or the floor with their hands. Actually, we should be hinging from the knees *and* hips and sitting our bums down towards the floor. That's why I really love the use of the chair here to help develop the technique of sitting down into the legs, rather than hunching over and using our backs to lift back up. What you are after here is both a knee hinge and a hip hinge – not one or the other alone. Try to keep the weight equal in the feet as you squat, too – no lifting the heels or the toes as you move.

Single leg balances to single calf raises

In phase 2, we will be introducing some impact into the exercises, and to help with this it's a good idea to start to develop your calf strength. Your calves can really help you to cope with impact, as they give you bounce and help to absorb impact forces. Single leg work is so important for helping to build pelvic stability and adds an extra core challenge, too.

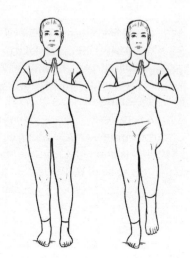

1. Start in a nice, neutral standing position, hands in prayer position at your chest.
2. Shift your weight over to your right leg, keeping the knee soft, but not bent.
3. Slowly start to lift your left foot away from the floor, putting all your body weight through your right leg. You can either leave your left tiptoes on the floor or completely lift the foot off the floor to balance.
4. Hold for up to 60 seconds (which is a lot, ok!) and then switch legs.

Progression – single calf raises

1. Start standing, feet hip-width apart and hands in prayer position.
2. Come up into a calf raise with both feet and find your balance.
3. Shift your weight over to your left foot as much as you feel safe doing so.
4. Inhale to lower the left heel to the floor and exhale to lift the left heel back up into a calf raise.
5. Repeat 10–12 times, then switch legs.

TIP: While yes, you are trying to put your weight through one leg here, try not to side bend, or overly lean or cause crazy changes to the rest of your posture as you do so. Ideally, stay as neutral as you can, and simply drive more weight down through one leg in this exercise.

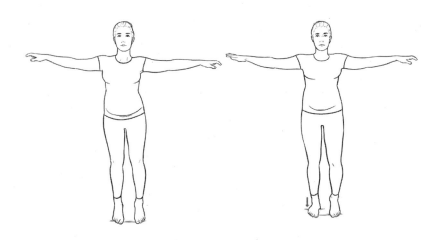

Example routines

Routine 1 combines all of the easier exercise options. Routine 2 combines the progressions. Feel free to repeat the routines to help you build up to the recommended 150 minutes of physical activity per week (an example week could be 5 x 30 minute workouts). You can mix these routines up, based on the versions that work best for you at present. You might choose the initial version for some exercises, and for others the progression. Listen to your body and do whatever feels right for you, right now.

Routine 1

- Pelvic tilts
- Zips
- Head unweighting
- Knee folds
- Mini hip hinges
- Static baby lunges
- Mini squats
- Single leg balances

Routine 2 (the progressions)

- Hip rolls
- Knee lifts
- Ab prep
- Single leg extensions
- Full hip hinges
- Full lunges
- Full squats
- Single calf raises

Your pelvic floor exercise

Spaghetti

As a Pilates teacher, I find myself using all manner of cues to encourage clients to target the right muscles. I am a big fan of visualisations as cues, and the fact I'm an ex-chef might explain why there are so many food-related ones.

In this visualisation, you will imagine that you are sucking spaghetti off the floor with your pelvic floor. This will encourage you to squeeze and lift it, which is key for good engagement. If it feels too weird, feel free to swap it for another imaginary prop – some people prefer to imagine sucking in a tampon or drawing up a piece of thread. What is key here is that it works for you.

Remember that a pelvic floor workout includes ten slow holds and ten fast pulses (see p. 68 for more on this). This exercise is aimed at encouraging good technique, so use it to really nail your pelvic floor contractions – but don't forget to keep practising your full pelvic floor workouts too.

1. Start in a comfortable position – this might be seated, lying, side-lying, standing.
2. Close your eyes (this will help you to focus internally) and try to clear your mind.
3. Focus on your breathing by bringing your awareness to breathing in and out through your nose. Relax your jaw and ensure your tongue is relaxed in your mouth.
4. Inhale to prepare and, as you exhale, imagine sucking up a piece of spaghetti with your vagina.
5. Inhale to release and imagine it being removed, then exhale to repeat.
6. Repeat 8–10 times.

TIP: When you get a good pelvic floor contraction, your perineum will move due to the tightening of the surrounding area (the perineum is the tissue between the vaginal opening and the anus). If you are in any doubt as to whether you are activating your pelvic floor, you could try the following during a pelvic floor exercise:

- Use a mirror to watch the perineum and see if you notice it ascend and descend as the pelvic floor moves.
- Place a clean finger on the perineum to feel if it moves.
- Insert a clean finger inside the vagina and feel for a tightening of the vaginal wall on a pelvic floor contraction.

So there you have it – postnatal phase 1. I hope you've found it helpful, and it's given you the confidence to reintroduce some of the movements you haven't managed for a while or that felt a little scary at first. Remember that your body goes through a lot during pregnancy and labour, but it is also incredibly clever, adaptable and resilient – it just needs a bit of care and attention along the way. Whatever stage you're at in your postnatal journey (4 weeks, 4 months, 4 years . . .) things do get better, and you will get stronger. So keep going.

If, however, something doesn't feel right, you just don't feel yourself or the exercises don't feel to you as I have described them, do seek help. It may be that you need to consult a pelvic health physiotherapist or that your GP simply has to check your scars. As parents, we tend to place ourselves so far down the priority list – but you matter, too!

Once you feel confident with all (or at least most) of the exercises in this phase and are ready to reintroduce some impact, you can move on to phase 2. There is always the option to go back to phase 1 if phase 2 doesn't feel right, or you can simply continue with phase 1, just adding in some phase 2 moves. It's totally up to you and how you feel. There is no rush, and there are no time frames to stick to when working through this book. As I keep saying, we are all different, so listen to *your* body and don't compare yourself to anyone else.

Postnatal phase 2

~~~~~~

Hooray, you've made it to phase 2! This is where you start to build on what you have learned in the recovery phase and phase 1. It's ideal for those who feel ready to start adding in more advanced movements involving some impact (think jumping and bouncing around). I have heard too many women joke that they'll never use a trampoline again because they have had children, and I'm not standing for that! Trampolines are far too much fun to miss out on, so let's learn to cope with (and enjoy) some impact.

What will we be covering?

This is an exciting time, and an important process if you want the freedom to be able to run, jump, skip, trampoline or skydive (yes, I have had clients whose postnatal goal was to return to the skies as soon as possible). Being able to manage impact allows you to try new things, or return to old things, without worrying that your insides are going to fall out (a genuine concern I hear) or that you'll do something that may harm you.

If you've read Part 1, you'll understand the difference between musculoskeletal and cardiovascular exercises, and why they are both so important (if not, you should skip back to pp. 14–15 now.). In phase 1, we introduced exercises that were focused on musculoskeletal strengthening, meaning they were building up your muscle and joint strength. Now we want to add focus to your cardiovascular strength (your heart, veins and arteries), as well as continuing with your exercises from phase 1, if you wish.

Introducing impact back into your training, in my eyes, is really morale-boosting. For me, it marked the realisation that I'd regained some confidence in my body, I no longer felt fragile or broken and I was ready to start pushing myself a little harder. As someone who has spent a lifetime interested in sport and fitness, this was important to me and my mental health. You may not have *exactly* the same feelings, but please know that this phase is a real marker for progress. You have worked hard to get to this point, and you deserve to enjoy whatever movement you add in now.

Essentially, the aim of this phase is to test how impact *feels* for your body, learn how to cope with it and get better at managing it or using it to your advantage.

What do I need to know?

So I've spoken a lot about reintroducing impact. But what do I actually mean by impact – and why bother reintroducing it?

Imagine a form of physical activity, such as running: what happens to the rest of the body when your feet hit the floor on each stride? You can be the best runner in the world, with the smoothest technique, but there's no denying that you are going to experience the force of your bodyweight when your feet hit the tarmac. This is called impact.

Now, how your body deals with that impact is important. You want to be able to absorb it, cope with it and, ultimately, use it to help push you off into your next stride. What you don't want is to leak urine when you land, lose control and stability in your ankles or fall over or stumble with each step. These are very extreme examples of someone who cannot manage the impact of running very well, but if even one of those issues arose, it would make this form of movement either unsafe or unenjoyable. And that's not what you want.

So in this phase, we will gradually reintroduce impact to see how you are currently managing it (because maybe you haven't done anything involving impact since pre-conception) and then build your strength up to cope with increasing levels.

It (almost) goes without saying, then, that if you haven't already, I would really like you to familiarise yourself with the concept of pressure management (see p. 174). This will help you to assess how the increase in impact is affecting your core, and if you need to regress or progress an exercise to make it work for you.

Please ensure that any labour scars you have (Caesarean or vaginal) are well healed and you no longer have any pain or tenderness around the areas in question. Should any of the exercises in this phase cause them to become sore, stick with the easier version or cease the exercise altogether and move back to phase 1 for now.

If you haven't already got a supportive sports bra, please, *please* do get your hands on one now. No matter how postnatal you are, the ligaments of the breasts are important, and a good sports bra will protect them so much better than your old pre-conception ones, especially when you start adding in the impact.

So with all this in mind, let's get started with the exercises. You'll see that, just like in phase 1, I have listed movements that are actually two exercises in one. Each starts with the easiest version, for those who are just entering phase 2, and then shows you the more advanced option to build up to.

The following exercises are mainly cardiovascular focused, but they will also, of course, strengthen the musculoskeletal system. You have the option of slowing them right down and focusing more on the technique and strength aspects or speeding them up and building on your cardiovascular strength. I have stated how long each exercise should be done for, but please feel free to adapt – remember, as ever, that everyone will be at different stages of the postnatal journey.

As the exercises here have a cardiovascular effect on the body, I would recommend starting with the warm-up from pp. 74–76 and making use of the cool-down on pp. 87–88 at the end of your workouts, too. In between, you could do each of the below exercises in order, one after another with no break, or do each one followed by a 30-second rest. You'll find some sample routines at the end of this chapter.

Your exercises: phase 2

Now that you're getting used to moving your body again, let's get into the exercises you'll be doing in postnatal phase 2.

Do remember that for each exercise there is an easier option to start with, and a progression to build up to as you get stronger and feel ready.

Marching on the spot to straight-leg bouncing

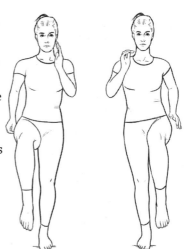

Marching on the spot is a nice, gentle way of introducing some cardiovascular challenge, without adding much impact – and you can adapt how fast you move with it. Eventually, you might increase the speed, until you're jogging or even running on the spot. Straight-leg bouncing is a great running drill that feels silly (just a heads-up on that one) but gives you an idea of what running impact will feel like, and tests how your body copes with it. It's a really simple exercise.

1. Start standing and slowly begin to pick up your feet, as though walking or marching on the spot. Make sure you're moving your arms, too, as the more you move them, the bigger the cardiovascular challenge.
2. Pick up to a pace that challenges you.
3. Repeat for 30–60 seconds.

Progression – straight-leg bouncing

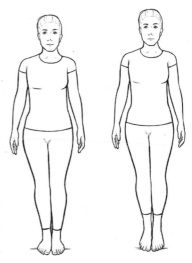

1. Start standing, legs together, arms wherever they feel comfortable (I let mine dangle by my sides).
2. Keeping the legs together and straight, start to bounce on the spot, as fast as feels manageable for you. Allow the knees to be soft to absorb some of the impact.
3. Repeat for 30–60 seconds.

TIP: For the straight-leg bouncing, yes, you want to absorb *some* of the impact (because it's a good skill to learn), but you also want to *allow* some of it, so you can test out how that feels on the body. How does your pelvic floor feel? How does your core feel? It's a great way to build up to the impact created when running.

Lunge kicks to runner's lunges

These exercises also appear on pp. 160 (lunge kicks) and 163 (runner's lunges), but they're brilliant here, too, because many of us will have phased them out during pregnancy (they can get too challenging by the end), so we want to phase them back in when we can. I'm a massive fan of runner's lunges once mastered, but there's no denying that they are tricky and wobbly. They are a really good way to build lower body strength, plus bounce and stability – all great skills for impact. Take your time, though, and nail your lunge technique.

1. Start in a standing position, feet hip-width apart, hands in prayer position and with a neutral spine.
2. Step the left leg back behind you, bend both knees into a lunge position and lean forwards just enough to maintain a neutral spine.

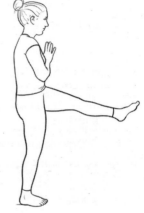
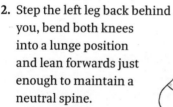
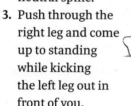
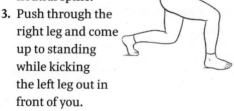

3. Push through the right leg and come up to standing while kicking the left leg out in front of you.
4. Repeat for 30–60 seconds, then swap legs.

Progression – runner's lunges

1. Start standing, with feet hip-width apart, hands in prayer position and a neutral spine.
2. Lunge back with your right leg, bending both knees and leaning forwards slightly.
3. Push yourself back up to standing and, as you do so, bring your right knee up and through towards your chest, while jumping up using your left leg.

4. Land as softly as you can on your left foot and take your right leg back into a lunge again, ready to go again.

5. Repeat for 30–60 seconds and then swap legs.

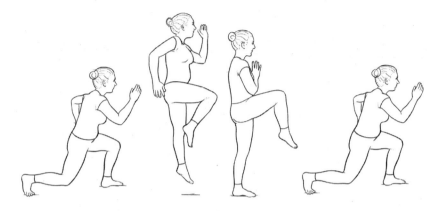

TIP: Both of these exercises are wobbly, so feel free to stand near a wall or hold the back of a chair. Even if you are aiming for a cardiovascular effect, you do not need to do these super speedily. You're using big, global muscles that require a lot of energy, so you'll find your heart rate increases, even at a slower speed.

Squat calf raises to squat jumps

Squats are an easy and effective way of raising your heart rate, and adding in some extra calf activation will really help you to manage impact in other areas (the calves help to propel you forwards, but also play a major role in shock absorption). Both of these exercises include calf activation, but squat jumps introduce impact, too.

1. Start in your chosen squat position (parallel feet hip-width apart or sumo squat position with feet wider than hip-width apart and in turnout). Bend your knees and sit down into a squat.
2. Stand up, and once your legs are straight, lift both heels to come into a calf raise.
3. Repeat for 30–60 seconds.

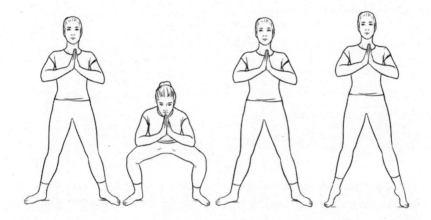

Progression – squat jumps

1. Start in the same position as above.
2. Squat down, but as you come back up to standing, jump into the air, landing as softly as you can and lowering back down into a squat.
3. Repeat for 30–60 seconds.

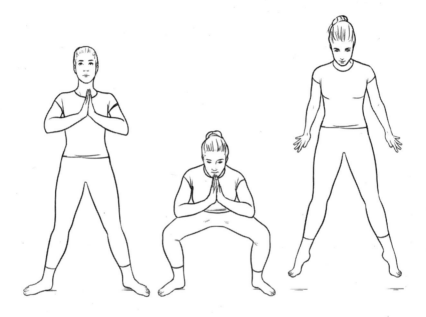

TIP: Find the squat position that works best for you in these exercises. If your pelvic floor is struggling with impact (or it's still rebuilding its strength), you may find that sumo squat position (where the legs are wide and in turnout) is harder, and that feet hip-width apart and parallel might be more manageable.

Jogging on the spot to sprinting

A really simple drill for running, as you
are literally practising technique and
testing impact, but on the spot.

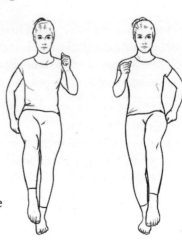

1. I would always start with some
   walking on the spot here for a few
   seconds at least.
2. Build up to jogging on the spot,
   ensuring the arms are moving,
   too, as this will increase the
   cardiovascular load and encourage
   good running technique.
3. Repeat for 30–60 seconds.

Progression – sprinting

1. Start by jogging on the spot for at least a few seconds.
2. Build up to sprinting, not forgetting to allow the arms to move freely
   here, too.
3. Repeat for 30–60 seconds.

TIP: Play around with the impact here. Even if you *can* be very light on
your feet, it can be worth allowing some impact. This is because when you
get tired on actual runs, you won't be able to be as light as you can be
when practising on the spot. So it's important you've tested out what
slightly heavier footwork would feel like, ahead of time.

Low-impact jacks to full jacks

You can guarantee that any cardiovascular class you attend in the future will include jumping jacks, and they can be tricky for the pelvic floor if it's still recovering, as you're landing with the legs apart, with impact. Here, you can start with no impact and build up gradually.

1. Start standing, arms by your sides, elbows soft, palms resting on legs, feet together.
2. Tap one foot out to the side as you take both arms overhead, then bring the leg in as the arms come down.
3. Take the other leg out to the side and tap the floor as the arms go overhead, and then bring it all back in.
4. Repeat for 30–60 seconds.

Progression – full jacks

1. Start in the same position as step 1 above.
2. Jump up and land with both feet hip-width apart and arms overhead, before jumping back to your start position.
3. Repeat for 30–60 seconds.

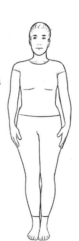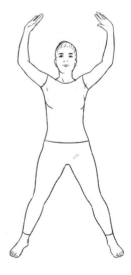

TIP: Think about landing as softly as possible for the full jacks, and while it's harder, it'll teach you great shock absorption for other activities.

Grapevines to skaters

I love grapevines. They remind me of old-school aerobics or step classes I used to attend – and they're low impact. Skaters kick it up a notch and are a dynamic movement, making them a great challenge.

1. Stand at the right end of your mat.
2. Step your left leg to the left, open your arms out to crucifix position, then, as you step your right leg in to join the left, lower the arms back down.
3. Repeat, and this should bring you to the other end of your mat (the left end), ready to then reverse the move and take two steps back to the right end of your mat.
4. Repeat for 30–60 seconds.

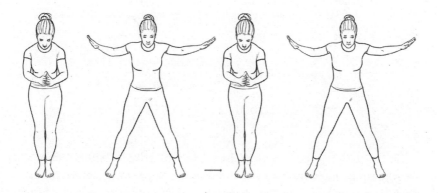

Progression – skaters

1. Stand at the right end of your mat.
2. Leap towards the left end of your mat, extending your arms out wide and landing as softly as you can on your left leg, taking your right foot out behind you like a tail.
3. Leap to the right-hand side of your mat, landing on your right leg and taking your left foot out behind you like a tail.
4. Repeat for 30–60 seconds.

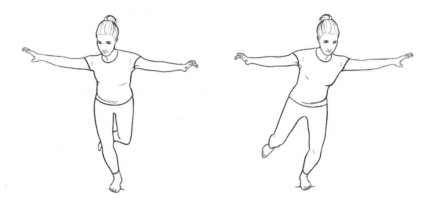

TIP: Skaters are meant to be explosive, so really think about dropping low, jumping high, then dropping low again, as you land. You want them to feel springy and light, but obviously, at first, they may feel quite heavy and loud, so take your time and build up gradually.

Low-impact split punches to full split punches

I swear this is more of a test of your mind than your fitness, especially if you're tired, as it only feels right if you have the opposite arm and leg out in front of you. It may take a few attempts.

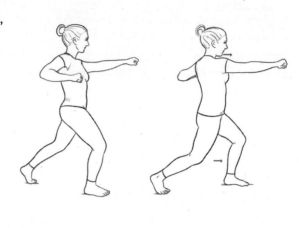

1. Stand with feet hip-width apart, hands at your chest in fists, as if ready for a fight.
2. Take your left foot and tap it out in front of you, while taking your right arm and punching it forwards.
3. Bring the leg and arm back in, and switch to repeat with the right foot and left arm.
4. Repeat for 30–60 seconds.

Progression – full split punches

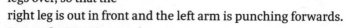

1. Stand with feet hip-width apart, left leg out slightly in front and right arm in front in a punching position.
2. Jump up and swap the legs over, so that the right leg is out in front and the left arm is punching forwards.
3. Repeat for 30–60 seconds.

TIP: Feel free to add some weights in your hands here to increase the effort, while not necessarily increasing the impact. Land as softly as you can, with both feet at the same time on the full split punch.

Example routines

Below, you'll find two example routines. Routine 1 combines all of the easier exercise options. Routine 2 combines the progressions with a rest period (which you do not have to utilise). Feel free to repeat the routines to help you build up to the recommended 150 minutes of physical activity per week (an example week could be 5 x 30 minute workouts). You can mix these routines up, based on the versions that work best for you at present. Listen to your body and do whatever feels right for you, right now.

Routine 1

- *Warm-up*
- Marching on the spot
- Lunge kicks
- Squat calf raises
- Jogging on the spot
- Low-impact jacks
- Grapevines
- Low-impact split punch
- Repeat for 2–3 sets
- *Cool-down*

Routine 2 (the progressions)

- *Warm-up*
- Straight-leg bouncing
- 30-second rest
- Runner's lunges
- 30-second rest
- Squat jumps

- 30-second rest
- Sprinting
- 30-second rest
- Full jacks
- 30-second rest
- Skaters
- 30-second rest
- Full split punches
- Repeat for 2-3 sets
- *Cool-down*

Your pelvic floor exercise

Staggered lifts

When it comes to pelvic floor exercises, it's really tempting to do them all sitting down, legs crossed, eyes closed, totally focused (baby asleep or entertained). And yes, there really is a place for that – being mindful is key, and practising them in this way is the easiest option, so will help you to nail your technique. But you won't always cough or sneeze (or create pressure in your core) while sitting cross-legged, focusing on your pelvic floor. You might be running for a bus, lunging to stop your child falling over or jumping on a trampoline. So it's time to start being creative with your pelvic floor exercises and challenge yourself in other positions.

1. Stand with feet hip-width apart.
2. Imagine you are standing in the middle of a clockface, with the number twelve ahead of you.
3. Step your right foot out to 2pm on your imaginary clockface. This will create a sort of staggered foot position – awkward, but very functional.
4. Put one hand on your tummy, and the other on one of your bum cheeks.
5. Inhale to prepare and then, as you exhale, lift your pelvic floor and hold for 8–10 seconds.
6. Repeat these slow holds 5 times.

7. Now practise 5 fast pulses. (You might feel your lower tummy contract as you do this but try not to clench your bum cheek.)
8. Come back to your start position and then take your left foot out to 10pm on your imaginary clockface.
9. Repeat your 5 slow holds and your 5 fast pulses.
10. Rest.

TIP: Placing your hands on your body for feedback can be really helpful here, as it's tempting to cheat and 'muscle through' an exercise when you make it harder. Here, you'll be able to feel if you clench your bum cheek (a sign you're cheating). If this happens, try to reduce the amount of effort you put in initially, until the bum cheek calms down, and think about the muscle engagement as being more internal (maybe imagine sucking up a tampon or gripping a finger with your vagina).

So that's it. Phase 2 – a reintroduction to impact, and hopefully a step closer to feeling a little more like you! I hope you've loved getting your body moving more and that you've also felt an increase in confidence as you continue to challenge it. You might repeat phase 2 for weeks, or even months, until you feel ready to move back to the movements you did pre-conception, but hopefully, with time, you'll feel safe running, jumping, climbing, tackling . . . whatever movement makes you happy.

When you feel ready to reintroduce other forms of training, keep in mind what you have learned about pressure management and movement technique, and you will be in a far safer position. You can always regress exercises if you need to or move back into phase 2 if you realise you're not quite ready for pre-conception fitness yet. And overall, keep in mind the CMOs' guidelines for postnatal women (see p. 254) and aim to get back to their recommendations when you can, if you haven't already.

Conclusion

As I sit here writing, now 4 weeks after my son Kit's birth, I am reminded yet again of how incredible our bodies are, and how resilient and powerful we can be. Conception, pregnancy and birth are monumental challenges, yet we face them head on and get the job done. You should be beyond proud of yourself, and I hope you feel like an absolute badass having navigated this journey! Well done, us. (I realise this may sound patronising, but so often we think of the things we haven't managed to do, or haven't done very well, and forget to praise ourselves for just how much we have achieved and overcome.)

On that note, I really hope that this book has helped you through this challenging period and has given you the confidence to move your body in a way that feels good for you, at a time when it's all too easy to doubt every decision you make. My dream is that every pregnant person who wants to stay active reads this book, and feels supported in moving their body, reassured as to the safety and benefit of an active pregnancy.

If you've made it to the end of phase 2 and are ready to fly the exercise nest and move back into pre-conception training, I am so very proud of you! To juggle the postnatal period and carve out time to rehabilitate your body is tough, and I hope it's been an enjoyable experience. Now you know the exercises in these pages inside out, there is no reason you can't use them for life. (I still use them *years* after having Freya.) Everything you've learned here will help to keep your body functional, strong, powerful and, hopefully, injury free, so do keep the book to hand and dip in and out when you need to.

Going forwards, no matter what method of movement you choose, please can I ask that you continue to put your body's performance and function first. It can be so easy to be swept away with the fitness industry's promises and the advertising campaigns for dieting and food fads, and to see physical activity as a way of controlling how your body looks.

But your body is about so much more than the way it looks, how much it weighs, or what dress size you fit into. *You* are so much more than your body, and it doesn't define you. Try to avoid putting movement and superficial gains in the same category and instead see movement as being a bringer of joy, a stepping stone towards improved health, a great way to meet other people and something you are choosing (rather than having) to do.

Finally, thank you for being part of The Bump Plan community, and for sharing this journey with me. You will never know how much each of you means to me, and how lucky I feel that I get to work with people like you, every day.

Acknowledgements

~~~~~~

In a strange way this has been the hardest part of the book to write, and I have stared at this page for longer than I care to admit. This is not because I can't think of who to thank, but because there have been so many people who have touched my working and personal life that have led me to where I am now – there's simply too many to list.

However, there are some seriously important people whom this book really wouldn't be here without!

Thank you to: The incredible women in the pre- and postnatal field, who are helping to raise awareness, drive important research, and improve standards for women's fitness, who have inspired me more than they will ever know. Perhaps most notably the founders of the Active Pregnancy Foundation, Sally and Marlize, whose endless passion has had a drastically positive effect on the industry! Marlize's inbox will no doubt be grateful when this book is finished and I cannot thank her enough for her input, her patience, her knowledge and her support. What a woman!

Margie Davenport, Grainne Donnelly and Emma Brockwell – strong, inspiring women who have heavily influenced my work, and in various ways helped make The Bump Plan what it is. They will not realise the level of their input – but I do!

My editor, Cyan at HarperCollins, for her belief in this book from the very beginning, and her patience and kindness throughout the process. Working with an author who is heavily pregnant can't have been easy, but she never let it show. As a fellow mother, previous Bump Plan client, and the kindest soul, I couldn't have asked for a better editor. To the wider HarperCollins team, thank you for helping me bring this book baby into the world.

My agent Jonathan, who repeatedly gives me the confidence that I am an actual author, and can write a whole freaking book.

My amazing PA Charlotte, who held the fort and kept a rapidly growing business in check while I wrote the book, while growing a child, while relocating my family 100 miles away, and while generally juggling many balls. Her positivity and support, while also navigating the loss of her beautiful son Zander, will never be forgotten.

My wonderful family, who always encourage me to "go for it", and for never doubting me, when I doubt myself. To my daughter Freya – the original Bump in the Bump Plan and the reason I work as hard as I do so that hopefully her generation will have a better relationship with their bodies. To my son Kit for staying in my womb for as long as you did, so I could finish the book – what a legend. And to my husband who works as hard on The Bump Plan as I do, while sharing parenting equally with me, but never wants recognition (he'll hate this mention).

The amazing experts who selflessly shared their knowledge for the book, and who have helped support The Bump Plan in its development over the years. I feel so lucky to work in an industry with so many incredible minds, who simply want women's experiences to be improved.

And finally, and perhaps most importantly, to every single Bump Plan member over the last few years who have made me love my job, every day. I will never stop pinching myself that I get to do what I do, and they will never know just how privileged I feel to be part of their journeys.

Sources

Introduction

1. UK Chief Medical Officers' Physical Activity Guidelines 2019 and Ming W.K., Ding W., Zhang C.J.P., Zhong L., Long Y., Li Z., Sun C., Wu Y., Chen H., Chen H., Wang Z. The effect of exercise during pregnancy on gestational diabetes mellitus in normal-weight women: a systematic review and meta-analysis. *BMC Pregnancy Childbirth.* 2018 Nov 12;18(1):440. doi: 10.1186/s12884-018-2068-7. PMID: 30419848; PMCID: PMC6233372.

2. Daley A.J., Foster L., Long G., Palmer C., Robinson O., Walmsley H., Ward R. The effectiveness of exercise for the prevention and treatment of antenatal depression: systematic review with meta-analysis. *BJOG: An International Journal of Obstetrics & Gynaecology.* 2015 Jan;122(1):57-62. doi: 10.1111/1471-0528.12909. Epub 2014 Jun 17. PMID: 24935560.

3. Eclarinal J.D., Zhu S., Baker M.S., Piyarathna D.B., Coarfa C., Fiorotto M.L., Waterland R.A. Maternal exercise during pregnancy promotes physical activity in adult offspring. *The FASEB Journal.* 2016 Jul;30(7): 2541-8. doi: 10.1096/fj.201500018R. Epub 2016 Mar 31. PMID: 27033262; PMCID: PMC4904289.

4. Davenport M.H., Meah V.L., Ruchat S.M., Davies G.A., Skow R.J., Barrowman N., Adamo K.B., Poitras V.J., Gray C.E., Jaramillo Garcia A.,

Sobierajski F., Riske L., James M., Kathol A.J., Nuspl M., Marchand A.A., Nagpal T.S., Slater L.G., Weeks A., Barakat R., Mottola M.F. Impact of prenatal exercise on neonatal and childhood outcomes: a systematic review and meta-analysis. *British Journal of Sports Medicine.* 2018 Nov;52(21):1386-1396. doi: 10.1136/bjsports -2018-099836. PMID: 30337465.
5. The Active Pregnancy Foundation Annual Survey 2022.

Part 1: What You Need to Know

1. UK Chief Medical Officers' Physical Activity Guidelines 2019. https:// assets.publishing.service.gov.uk/government/uploads/system /uploads/attachment_data/file/832868/uk-chief-medical-officers -physical-activity-guidelines.pdf
2. Ibid.
3. Public Health England. Guidance Health Matters: physical activity – prevention and management of long-term conditions. https://www.gov .uk/government/publications/health-matters-physical-activity /health-matters-physical-activity-prevention-and-management-of -long-term-conditions
4. Ibid.
5. Caspersen C.J., Powell K.E., Christenson G.M. Physical activity, exercise, and physical fitness: definitions and distinctions for health-related research. *Public Health Report.* 1985 Mar-Apr;100(2):126-31. PMID: 3920711; PMCID: PMC1424733 and with further input and clarification by Dr Marlize De Vivo.
6. The Fertility Society of Australia. The role of exercise in improving fertility, quality of life and emotional well-being. https://www .fertilitysociety.com.au/wp-content/uploads/FSA-The-role-of-exercise -in-improving-fertility-2016.pdf

7. Prosen M., Zvanut B., Pucer P., Mivšek A.P., Petrocnik P., Tuomi J. The importance of physical activity in improving preconception health: a scoping review. *Kontakt.* 2021 Dec;23(4):247-255. doi: 10.32725 /kont.2021.051

8. Wise L.A., Rothman K.J., Mikkelsen E.M., Sørensen H.T., Riis A.H., Hatch E.E. A prospective cohort study of physical activity and time to pregnancy. *Fertility and Sterility.* 2012 May;97(5):1136-1142. doi: 10.1016/j .fertnstert.2012.02.025. Epub 2012 Mar 15.

9. NHS Overview Infertility. https://www.nhs.uk/conditions/infertility/

10. UK Chief Medical Officers' Physical Activity Guidelines 2019. https://assets.publishing.service.gov.uk/government/uploads/system /uploads/attachment_data/file/832868/uk-chief-medical-officers -physical-activity-guidelines.pdf

11. UK Chief Medical Officers' Physical Activity Guidelines 2019. https:// assets.publishing.service.gov.uk/government/uploads/system /uploads/attachment_data/file/832868/uk-chief-medical-officers -physical-activity-guidelines.pdf

12. The American College of Obstetricians and Gynecologists. Physical activity and exercise during pregnancy and the postpartum period. https://www.acog.org/clinical/clinical-guidance/committee-opinion /articles/2020/04/physical-activity-and-exercise-during-pregnancy -and-the-postpartum-period

13. Davenport M.H., Davies G.A., Meah V.L. Why can't I exercise during pregnancy? Time to revisit medical 'absolute' and 'relative' contraindications: systematic review of evidence of harm and a call to action. *British Journal of Sports Medicine.* 2020 Dec;54(23):1395-1404. doi: 10.1136 /bjsports-2020-102042. PMID: 32513676.

14. UK Chief Medical Officers' Physical Activity Guidelines 2019. https://assets.publishing.service.gov.uk/government/uploads/system /uploads/attachment_data/file/832868/uk-chief-medical-officers -physical-activity-guidelines.pdf

15. Sanghavi M., Rutherford J.D. Cardiovascular physiology of pregnancy. *Circulation*. 2014 Sept;130(12):1003-1008. doi: 10.1161/CIRCU LATIONAHA.114.009029

16. Soma-Pillay P., Nelson-Piercy C., Tolppanen H., Mebazaa A. Physiological changes in pregnancy. *Cardiovascular Journal of Africa*. 2016 Mar-Apr;27(2):89-94. doi: 10.5830/CVJA-2016-021. PMID: 27213856; PMCID: PMC4928162.

17. Sanghavi M., Rutherford J.D. Cardiovascular physiology of pregnancy. *Circulation*. 2014 Sept;130(12):1003-1008. doi: 10.1161/CIRCULATIONAHA .114.009029

18. Fernandes da Mota P.G., Pascoal A.G., Carita A.I., Bø K. Prevalence and risk factors of diastasis recti abdominis from late pregnancy to 6 months postpartum, and relationship with lumbo-pelvic pain. *Manual Therapy*. 2015 Feb;20(1):200-5. doi: 10.1016/j.math.2014.09.002. Epub 2014 Sep 19. PMID: 25282439.

19. Sperstad J.B., Tennfjord M.K., Hilde G., Ellström-Engh M., Bø K. Diastasis recti abdominis during pregnancy and 12 months after childbirth: prevalence, risk factors and report of lumbopelvic pain. *British Journal of Sports Medicine*. 2016 Sep;50(17):1092-6. doi: 10.1136/ bjsports-2016-096065. Epub 2016 Jun 20. PMID: 27324871; PMCID: PMC5013086.

Part 2: Your Conception and Pregnancy Workouts

1. UK Chief Medical Officers' Physical Activity Guidelines 2019. https:// assets.publishing.service.gov.uk/government/uploads/system /uploads/attachment_data/file/832868/uk-chief-medical-officers -physical-activity-guidelines.pdf

2. Ibid.

3. NICE [was published February 2013, updated September 2017]. Fertility problems: assessment and treatment. Clinical guideline [CG156]. Last updated: September 2017. https://www.nice.org.uk/guidance /cg156/resources/fertility-problems-assessment-and-treatment -pdf-35109634660549

4. HFEA (May 2019). Fertility treatment 2019 [most up-to-date report]: trends and figures. https://www.hfea.gov.uk/about-us/publications /research-and-data/fertility-treatment-2019-trends-and-figures/

5. Hardefeldt P.J., Penninkilampi R., Edirimanne S., Eslick G.D. Physical Activity and Weight Loss Reduce the Risk of Breast Cancer: A Meta-analysis of 139 Prospective and Retrospective Studies. *Clinical Breast Cancer.* 2017 Oct;18(4):e601-e612. https://doi.org/10.1016/j.clbc.2017.10.010

6. Morris S.N., Missmer S.A., Cramer D.W., Powers R.D., McShane P.M., Hornstein M.D. Effects of Lifetime Exercise on the Outcome of In Vitro Fertilization. *Obstetrics & Gynecology.* 2006 Oct;108(4):938–945. doi:10.1097/01.AOG.0000235704.45652.0b. PMID: 17012457.

7. Morris S.N., Missmer S.A., Cramer D.W., Vitonis A.F., Hornstein M.D. Effects of exercise on in vitro fertilization (IVF) outcomes. *Fertility and Sterility.* 2004 Sept;82:S131. https://doi.org/10.1016/j.fertnstert.2004 .07.330

8. Domar A.D., Conboy L., Denardo-Roney J., Rooney K.L. Lifestyle behaviors in women undergoing invitro fertilization: a prospective study. *Fertility and Sterility.* 2012 Mar; 97:697-701.e1. https://doi.org/10 .1016/j.fertnstert.2011.12.012

9. Kucuk M., Doymaz F., Urman B. Assessment of the physical activity behavior and beliefs of infertile women during assisted reproductive technology treatment. *International Journal of Gynecology and Obstetrics.* 2010 Feb;108(2):132–134. https://doi.org/10.1016/j.ijgo.2009.08.036

10. Su T.J., Chen Y.C., Yang Y.S. Comparative study of daily activities of pregnant and non-pregnant women after in vitro fertilization and

embryo transfer. *Journal of the Formosan Medical Association.* 2001 Apr;100(4):262–268. PMID: 11393126.

11. Edwards R.G., Steptoe P.C., Purdy J.M. Establishing full-term human pregnancies using cleaving embryos grown in vitro. *BJOG: An International Journal of Obstetrics & Gynaecology.* 1980 Sept;87(9):737–756. https://doi.org/10.1111/j.1471-0528.1980.tb04610.x

12. Hawkins L.K., Rossi B.V., Correia K.F., Lipskind S.T., Hornstein M.D., Missmer S.A. Perceptions among infertile couples of lifestyle behaviors and in vitro fertilization (IVF) success. *Assisted Reproduction Technologies.* 2014 Mar;31:255–260. https://doi.org/10.1007/s10815-014-0176-5

13. Morris S.N., Missmer S.A., Cramer D.W., Powers D.R., McShane P.M., Hornstein M.D. Effects of Lifetime Exercise on the Outcome of In Vitro Fertilization. *Obstetrics & Gynecology.* 2006 Oct;108(4): 938–945. doi:10.1097/01.AOG.0000235704.45652.0b. PMID: 17012457.

14. Morris S.N., Missmer S.A., Cramer D.W., Vitonis A.F., Hornstein, M.D. Effects of exercise on in vitro fertilization (IVF) outcomes. *Fertility and Sterility.* 2004 Sept;82, S131. https://doi.org/10.1016/j.fertn stert.2004.07.330

15. Gaskins A.J., Williams P.L., Keller M.G., Souter I., Hauser R., Chavarro J.E. Maternal physical and sedentary activities in relation to reproductive outcomes following IVF. *Reproductive BioMedicine Online.* 2016 Oct;33(4):513–521. https://doi.org/10.1016/j.rbmo.2016.07.002

16. NHS guidance, Foods to Avoid in Pregnancy. https://www.nhs.uk /pregnancy/keeping-well/foods-to-avoid/

17. Ma X., Yue Z.-Q., Gong Z.-Q., Zhang H., Duan N.-Y., Shi Y.-T., Wei G.-X., Li Y.-F. The effect of diaphragmatic breathing on attention, negative affect and stress in healthy adults. *Frontiers in Psychology.* 2017 Jun 6;8:874. doi: 10.3389/fpsyg.2017.00874

18. Chen Y.-F., Huang X.-Y., Chien C.-H., Cheng J.-F. The effectiveness of diaphragmatic breathing relaxation training for reducing anxiety.

Perspectives in Psychiatric Care. 2017 Oct;53:329-336. https://doi.org /10.1111/ppc.12184

19. Hopper S.I., Murray S.L., Ferrara L.R., Singleton J.K. Effectiveness of diaphragmatic breathing for reducing physiological and psychological stress in adults: a quantitative systematic review. *JBI Database of Systematic Reviews and Implementation Reports*. 2019 Sept; 17(9):1855-1876 doi: 10.11124/JBISRIR-2017-003848

20. Wilcox A.J., Weinberg C.R., O'Connor J.F., Baird D.D., Schlatterer J.P., Canfield R.E., Armstrong E.G., Nisula B.C. Incidence of early loss of pregnancy. *The New England Journal of Medicine*. 1988 Jul 28;319(4):189-94. doi: 10.1056/NEJM198807283190401

21. Kim D.R., Wang E. Prevention of supine hypotensive syndrome in pregnant women treated with transcranial magnetic stimulation. *Psychiatry Research*. 2014 Aug 15;218(1-2):247-8. doi: 10.1016/j.psychres.2014.04.001. Epub 2014 Apr 12. PMID: 24768354; PMCID: PMC4057965.

22. The Royal College of Psychologists. Perinatal mental health services: recommendations for the provision of services for childbearing women. Sept 2021. https://www.rcpsych.ac.uk/docs/default-source/improving -care/better-mh-policy/college-reports/college-report-cr232---perinatal -mental-heath-services.pdf

23. National Childbirth Trust. Hidden Half campaign. https://www.nct .org.uk/get-involved/campaigns/hidden-half-campaign

24. NHS Talk Therapies for anxiety and depression. https://www .england.nhs.uk/mental-health/adults/nhs-talking-therapies/

25. Katonis P., Kampouroglou A., Aggelopoulos A., Kakavelakis K., Lykoudis S., Makrigiannakis A., Alpantaki K. Pregnancy-related low back pain. *Hippokratia*. 2011 Jul;15(3):205-10. PMID: 22435016; PMCID: PMC3306025.

26. Ashton-Miller J.A., Delancey J.O.L. On the biomechanics of vaginal birth and common sequelae. *Annual review of biomedical engineering*.

2009;11:163-76.   doi: 10.1146/annurev-bioeng-061008-124823.   PMID:
19591614; PMCID: PMC2897058.

27. Beckmann M.M., Stock O.M. Antenatal perineal massage for reduc-
ing perineal trauma. *The Cochrane Database of Systematic Reviews*. 2013;
Issue 4: Art. No.: CD005123. DOI: 10.1002/14651858.CD005123.pub3.
Accessed 13 February 2023.

Part 3: Your Postnatal Workouts

1. The Royal College of Obstetricians and Gynaecologists. Patient information leaflet: Assisted vaginal birth (ventouse or forceps). https://
www.rcog.org.uk/for-the-public/browse-all-patient-information
-leaflets/assisted-vaginal-birth-ventouse-or-forceps/

2. The Royal College of Obstetricians and Gynaecologists. Patient information leaflet: Perineal tears during childbirth. https://www.rcog.org
.uk/for-the-public/perineal-tears-and-episiotomies-in-childbirth
/perineal-tears-during-childbirth/

3. NHS Overview. Caesarean section. https://www.nhs.uk/conditions
/caesarean-section/

4. Fernandes da Mota P.G., Pascoal A.G., Carita A.I., Bø K. Prevalence
and risk factors of diastasis recti abdominis from late pregnancy to 6
months postpartum, and relationship with lumbo-pelvic pain. *Manual
Therapy*. 2015 Feb;20(1):200-5. doi: 10.1016/j.math.2014.09.002. Epub
2014 Sep 19. PMID: 25282439.

5. Sperstad J.B., Tennfjord M.K., Hilde G., Ellström-Engh M., Bø K.
Diastasis recti abdominis during pregnancy and 12 months after child-
birth: prevalence, risk factors and report of lumbopelvic pain. *British
Journal of Sports Medicine*. 2016 Sep;50(17):1092-6. doi: 10.1136/

bjsports-2016-096065. Epub 2016 Jun 20. PMID: 27324871; PMCID: PMC5013086.

6. Pelvic Obstetric and Gynaecological Physiotherapy. Vaginal prolapse: a guide for women. https://thepogp.co.uk/patient_information/womens _health/vaginal_prolapse.aspx

Resources

~~~~~~

When considering starting any exercise regime it can help to complete a pre-screening questionnaire that helps you understand if there is a health concern that needs guidance from your GP or health professional ahead of doing so.

Whilst these forms can never replace common sense, will never be able to screen for 100 per cent of conditions, and does not replace seeking medical advice, they can help flag any potential contraindications to exercise. If in doubt, please do speak to your GP.

The following Bump Plan pre-participation forms have been adapted from both the PAR-Q[1, 2] and the GAQ-P UK version[3], with extra input from Dr Marlize De Vivo, and the Active Pregnancy Foundation.

1. Chisholm D.M., Collis M.L., Kulak L.L., Davenport W., Gruber N. Physical activity readiness. *British Columbia Medical Journal* 17: 375–378, 1975.
2. Chisholm D.M., Collis M.L., Kulak L.L., Davenport W., Gruber N., Stewart G.W. PAR-Q validation report: the evaluation of a self-administered pre-exercise screening

questionnaire for adults. *Victoria: Canada: BC Ministry of Health and Health and Welfare 1978.*

3. A recent collaboration between the Canadian Society for Exercise Physiology (CSEP), the British Association of Sport and Exercise Sciences (BASES) and the Active Pregnancy Foundation has led to the creation of a UK version of CSEP's Get Active Questionnaire for Pregnancy.

The Bump Plan Trying to Conceive Pre-screening Form

Please answer each of the below questions honestly. Should you answer YES to any of the listed health conditions please ensure you talk with your doctor before you start your Bump Plan workouts, and together ensure you are both happy for you to take part.

Do you suffer from any of the following:	Yes	No
Heart or blood pressure problems		
Pains in the chest while exercising		
Epilepsy		
Diabetes		
Asthma or breathing difficulties		

Loss of your balance because of dizziness or loss of consciousness		
A bone or joint problem that could be made worse by a change in your physical activity		
Neck or back problems?		
Are you on any medication?		
Do you know of any reason you should not take part in cardiovascular and strength training?		
Are you currently undergoing IVF?		
Do you know of any other reason why you should not do physical activity?		

The Bump Plan Pregnancy Pre-screening Form

Please answer each of the below questions honestly. Should you answer YES to any of the listed health conditions please ensure you talk with your doctor before you start your Bump Plan workouts, and together ensure you are both happy for you to take part.

Do you suffer from any of the following:	Yes	No
Mild, moderate or severe respiratory diseases		
Mild, moderate or severe acquired or congenital heart disease		
Uncontrolled or severe arrhythmia		
Placental abruption		
Vasa previa		
Uncontrolled type 1 diabetes		
Intrauterine growth restriction (IUGR)		
Active preterm labour (i.e. regular and painful uterine contractions before 37 weeks of pregnancy) or preterm premature rupture of membranes (PPROMs)		

Pre-eclampsia		
Cervical insufficiency		
Placenta previa after 28 weeks		
Untreated thyroid disease		
Symptomatic, severe eating disorders		
Multiple nutrient deficiencies and/or chronic undernutrition		
Moderate—heavy smoking (>20 cigarettes per day) in the presence of comorbidities		
Twins (past 28 weeks pregnant) or are you expecting triplets or higher multiple births		
History of recurrent miscarriage		
Previous early delivery (pre 37 weeks)?		
Do you know of any other reason why you should not do physical activity?		

The Bump Plan Postnatal Pre-screening Form

Please answer each of the below questions honestly. Should you answer YES to any of the listed health conditions please ensure you talk with your doctor before you start your Bump Plan workouts, and together ensure you are both happy for you to take part.

General Health

Do any of these apply:	Yes	No
Has your doctor ever said that you have a heart condition and that you should only do physical activity recommended by a doctor?		
Do you feel pain in your chest when you do physical activity?		
In the past month, have you had chest pain when you were not doing physical activity?		
Do you lose balance because of dizziness, or do you ever lose consciousness?		
Do you have a bone or joint problem (for example, back, knee, hip) that could be made worse by a change in your physical activity?		

Is your doctor currently prescribing medication for your blood pressure or heart condition?		
Do you know of any other reason why you should not do physical activity?		

Postnatal Health

Please take a look at the list of symptoms below that can occur postnatally. For most women the below symptoms **do not** mean you **can't** engage in The Bump Plan Postnatal but given that everyone's circumstances and births are different you may wish to speak to your GP or birth provider **if you have any concerns** about whether you are ready to engage in postnatal exercise.

Pelvic girdle pain (PGP)

Carpal tunnel syndrome (wrist/finger/hand or forearm pain/ numbness or tingling)

Lack of total bladder/bowel control (urinary or faecal incontinence)

Piles/haemorrhoids/varicose veins/constipation

After effects of gestational diabetes

Joint pain

Vaginal disorder

Vaginal bleeding past the 6-week mark

Sacrum or sacroiliac joint pain (pain in the very low mid back – top of buttocks)

Knee pain (side/front)

Coccyx pain

Vaginal prolapse (cystocele, rectocele, uterine)

Rectal prolapse

Were you given an epidural during birthing?

C-Section wound discomfort or slow healing or ongoing
    numbness

Perineal scar pain, discharge from scar, or foul smell

Buttock/piriformis pain/sciatica

Acid reflux or digestion issues

Bleeding during or after exercise or any unexplained bleeding

Diastasis (separation of your abdominal muscles)

Breast health/breast feeding issues

Nerve damage during birthing (especially pudendal)

Anaemia or taking iron medication

Episiotomy cut, painful perineum or tears

Pelvic/abdominal cramps

Thrush (recently)